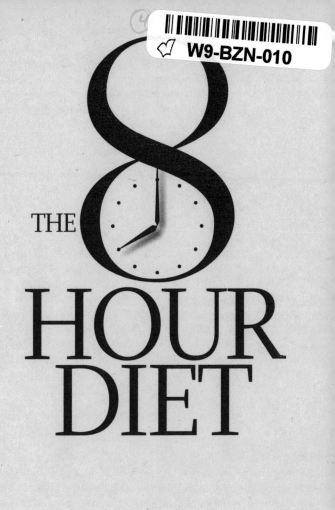

THE

HOUR
DIET

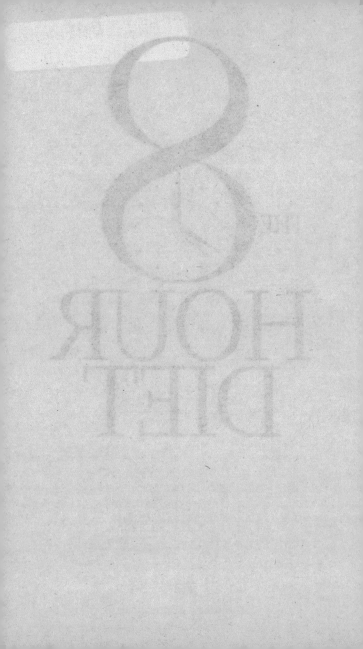

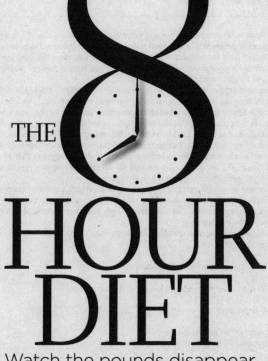

THE

8

HOUR
DIET

Watch the pounds disappear
without watching what you eat!

David Zinczenko
with Peter Moore, Editor of **Men'sHealth**.

St. Martin's Paperbacks

This book is intended as a reference volume only, not as a medical manual. The information given here is designed to help you make informed decisions about your health. It is not intended as a substitute for any treatment that may have been prescribed by your doctor. If you suspect that you have a medical problem, we urge you to seek competent medical help.

The information in this book is meant to supplement, not replace, proper exercise training. All forms of exercise pose some inherent risks. The editors and publisher advise readers to take full responsibility for their safety and know their limits. Before practicing the exercises in this book, be sure that your equipment is well-maintained, and do not take risks beyond your level of experience, aptitude, training, and fitness. The exercise and dietary programs in this book are not intended as a substitute for any exercise routine or dietary regimen that may have been prescribed by your doctor. As with all exercise and dietary programs, you should get your doctor's approval before beginning.

Mention of specific companies, organizations, or authorities in this book does not imply endorsement by the author or publisher, nor does mention of specific companies, organizations, or authorities imply that they endorse this book, its author, or the publisher.

Internet addresses and telephone numbers given in this book were accurate at the time it went to press.

Published by arrangement with Rodale Inc.

Men's Health is a registered trademark of Rodale Inc.

THE 8-HOUR DIET

Copyright © 2013 by Rodale Inc.
Photographs by Beth Bischoff.

All rights reserved.

For information address Rodale Inc., 733 Third Avenue, New York, NY 10010.

EAN: 978-1-250-06659-6

Printed in the United States of America

Rodale edition published 2013
St. Martin's Paperbacks edition / June 2015

St. Martin's Paperbacks are published by St. Martin's Press, 175 Fifth Avenue, New York, NY 10010.

10   9   8   7   6   5   4   3   2   1

*To future generations
of Americans.
May the obesity crisis
be something
they read about only
in history books.*

Contents

I want to tell you about a moment

that changed my life. Because it's going to change your life, too.

Several years ago, shortly after I was appointed editor in chief of *Men's Health*, I reached a personal crisis point. From the outside, my life seemed packed to perfection: I was taking high-powered breakfast meetings almost every day and wooing writers and photographers over dinners late at night. I was eating and working from sunup until long after sundown, but I was eating "healthy." And I was training like a maniac—running marathons on weekends and lifting weights at lunch several times a week. I needed all that food and all that exercise and all those early mornings and late nights to maintain the fitness and the workload that allowed me to be that *"Men's Health* guy."

I was the embodiment of "healthy and active." I was doing it all. And I was exhausted.

In 1999, my father died at age 52 of a stroke. It taught me two lessons. First, that life was short and I needed to cram everything I could into it. Second, that I needed to work out constantly and follow a strict diet to avoid the same fate. But after years of trying to do it all, I was just plain tired of being tired all the time. My doctor noted that I was also developing high blood pressure, just like my dad. Something inside me said that it was time to slow down. Maybe working so hard to be healthy wasn't so healthy, after all.

About the same time, I started reading some preliminary research about a new trend in weight-loss science that was yielding eye-opening results. One that didn't involve hard workouts, watching calories like a hawk, or pushing yourself and your body to the limit. It was a simple technique by which you cut down on the hours you spend eating, cut down on the intensity of exercise, and spend more time resting and enjoying the foods you love. Somewhere in the back of my mind, this new science started to take hold.

It wasn't a sudden decision, but over time I started skipping those power breakfast meetings. Instead, I took leisurely walks to work and just focused on getting things out of the way before tucking into a long, delicious lunch. I stopped working so hard in the gym, quit the marathons, fired the personal trainer. I started going to bed earlier instead of working so hard and "fueling" my body late into the night. And you know what happened?

No, I didn't gain weight. Just the opposite. Seven pounds in the first 10 days. I started losing weight and keeping it off, effortlessly, even as my blood pressure came under control. I was stunned.

I just thought this new plan would help me relax and enjoy life a little more.

I had no idea it would prove to be a weight-loss miracle.

I've been so inspired by how simple, easy, and enjoyable life has become that I've spent the last several years digging deeper into this research and boiling it down into an easy, accessible, life-altering plan. And the result is the book you hold in your hands. The 8-Hour Diet is the simplest, most sustainable weight-loss plan in the world. It will change your life. It will make you slimmer, healthier, and happier. It's worked for me.

I know it will work for you.

David Zinczenko

Acknowledgments

The ideas expressed in this book are, quite frankly, startling.

When we began researching the 8-Hour Diet, everything we thought we knew about eating to manage one's weight and improve one's health was turned on its head. As a result, we needed more than ever to do our homework, digging deeply into the science and relying on a network of reporters, researchers, fact checkers, and scientific advisors to see us safely, and wisely, through to the groundbreaking book you have in your hands.

In particular, we'd like to extend our thanks to Satchin Panda, PhD, associate professor of the regulatory biology laboratory at the Salk Institute in La Jolla, California, and Mark Mattson, PhD, chief of the Laboratory of Neurosciences at the National Institute on Aging, as well as their respective teams, for their revolutionary investigations into the health benefits of intermittent fasting. The leading theories and science in this field are theirs; the plan to implement it is ours.

To Maria Rodale and the Rodale family, whose dedication to pushing envelopes has left us anything but stationary! We thank them for empowering us to help people improve their lives and the world around them.

To George Karabatsos and his design crew, especially Mike Smith and Elizabeth Neal, who wrapped this revolution in an alluring package.

To Laura Roberson, Jordan Sward, Grant Stoddard, Lila Battis, Cathryne Keller, Theresa Dougherty, and Stephanie Smith, who also helped us bring this book to completion, in part by ignoring the concept of the 8-hour workday.

To our extraordinary *Eat This, Not That!* coauthor and friend Matt Goulding for whipping up more great recipes for this effort, and to BJ Gaddour for the heavy lifting that went into the cutting-edge exercise plan.

To Yelena Nesbit, Aly Mostel, Allison Keane, and Kateri Benjamin, who helped spread the word about this revolutionary plan.

To the Rodale Books team, especially Debbie McHugh, Steve Perrine, Chris Krogermeier, Jeff Csatari, Mike Zimmerman, Nancy Bailey, Beth Lamb, Bob Niegowski, Beth Bischoff, Ayla Christman, Adam Campbell, Michael Easter, and the Rodale production team. We appreciate your heroic efforts to bring this book to all who need it.

And now that you know all the people who worked so hard to bring this book to you, forget about them. We worked hard because we wanted weight loss to be easy for you—the person who really matters from this point forward.

Get ready to be amazed.

INTRODUCTION

THE 8-HOUR DIET

8 Hours to the Body You Want!

The simplest, most effective weight-loss plan ever invented

magine passing by a shop window, catching your reflection, and wondering—just for a moment—who that lean, attractive person is.

Then imagine discovering it's you.

Imagine the freedom that would come from being able to do whatever you want, eat whatever you want, and know—not think, not hope, but know for certain—that you'll never gain another pound.

Imagine never having to worry about your weight or its impact on your health, ever again.

If that sounds impossible, it's not. I know, because like tens of millions of Americans, I too have struggled with my weight. I know what it's like to be unhappy with my body, concerned about my heart health, stressed about my blood pressure and blood sugar, worried when the weather turned warmer that yet another embarassing swimsuit season was just around the corner. I know what it's like to shop for clothes, to pull some sizes that I hoped would fit, and yet find myself slinking home with a new pair of pants two, even three, sizes bigger than I'd expected.

Now I know that I'll never have to worry about gaining weight—even more important, all the health concerns that come with it—again. I know I have the secret to fast, permanent weight loss.

And that confidence is what I want for you.

The Secret of the 8-Hour Diet

When you think about the word "diet," you probably think of something that's confusing and hard to follow—and quite frankly, kind of depressing. You might think that seeing even the tiniest changes reflected in the mirror and on the bathroom scale will require sacrifice, deprivation, and a distinct absence of chocolate cake and barbecued ribs. Of course that's what you think because that's what you and I have been told a diet is. Weight loss is hard, right?

Wrong. You are about to read a weight-loss secret that is so simple, and yet so dramatically different from standard "diet" plans, that you'll swear it can't be true.

Losing weight just can't be this easy.

But it is. Indeed, over the next 300 pages, you're going to read eye-opening studies, life-altering expert insights, and remarkable personal tales of rapid, sustainable weight loss. Forget all the standard advice about cutting calories. Forget all the fad diets that limit your intake of this food or that food. Forget willpower, forget diet aids, forget counting calories, forget the glycemic index. Forget everything you have ever heard about weight loss, and instead, just do this:

Eat whatever you want, as much as you want.

But only eat during an 8-hour period each day (with a few cheats thrown in here and there!).

I know what you're thinking: If you're the skeptical, seen-it-all type like me, your b.s. meter is redlining like a college sophomore on a Monster bender. If it sounds too good to be true, it's probably not true. Right?

But the research is undeniable. Studies and experts from the most respected scientific organizations in the world— from the Salk Institute to the USDA to the University of California at Berkeley—keep coming to the same stunning, irrefutable finding: There *is* a magic bullet for weight loss.

Eat whatever you want, as much as you want.

But eat most of your food during an 8-hour period each day.

And the most remarkable thing of all: You only have to follow the diet 3 days a week. Three days a week!

Adhere to that advice, and you'll lose weight rapidly. (People who have tried this program report losing up to 20 pounds in just 6 weeks.) You'll dramatically slash your risk of heart disease, cancer, and diabetes. You'll improve your brain function and think more clearly and efficiently. You'll protect your body and mind against the effects of aging and stress. And you'll significantly extend your life expectancy.

All you need is 8 hours.

Lose Weight Like Never Before

The idea of eating as much as you want of any food you want—the idea that calories don't actually matter in the long run—goes against everything we've been told about losing weight. But then again, look at the evidence: More than two in every five Americans say they're currently on a diet. We spend more than $67 billion annually on diet books, weight-loss programs, and gym memberships. And yet two out of three American adults are overweight or obese. Obviously, what we've been told about losing weight is simply wrong, and all the diets we've been following are, in the end, wrong as well.

Well, that's about to change.

See, every other diet plan out there can be broken down into one of two types: calorie-restrictive diets and food-restrictive diets.

Calorie-restrictive diets are the most old-school, the kind that packed pantries of yore with rice cakes, cottage cheese, and Tab. As long as you ate fewer calories than your body burned each day, you'd lose weight. Science says that's the key to weight loss, after all.

But calorie-restrictive diets don't work, for the simple fact that we are what we are: quirky, fallible, human. Sure, maybe if you have the fortitude of Nelson Mandela, the endurance of Ryan Lochte, and the courage of Chesley "Sully" Sullenberger, you'll have no trouble passing up every hot, sticky Cinnabon that tickles your nostrils in the mall, every sizzling fajita that calls to you from a Red Robin, every stuffed-crust pizza that leaps out from the TV screen during a bowl game. But in the end, calorie-restrictive diets break down, because willpower breaks down, and the next thing you know, you're facedown in a package of Ding Dongs. In the long run, these traditional diets don't work.

The 8-Hour Diet is different because you can eat as many calories as you want. That's right: In a study conducted at the Beltsville Human Nutrition Research Center, scientists found that eating the same number of calories, just in a limited period of time, resulted in "a significant modification of body composition, including reductions in fat mass . . ."

Food-restrictive diets are the new-school way of losing weight. Eat all you want, just don't eat any carbs. Or fat. Or meat. Or dairy. Or high-glycemic foods. Or foods that Paleo men didn't eat. Or foods that aren't "whole." Or foods that have holes. From yogurt to yams to Yodels, someone some-

"IT MAKES ME FEEL PRETTY. BEAUTIFUL!"

Morgan lost 15 pounds in 6 weeks—and took control of her life

Morgan Jennings, 32, GATE CITY, VIRGINIA

OCCUPATION: **ACCOUNTANT**   HEIGHT: **5'4"**
STARTING WEIGHT: **192**   WEIGHT AFTER 6 WEEKS: **177**

When Morgan Jennings found out she was pregnant, she knew it was time to gear up and get healthy once and for all. But as a single mother who breastfeeds, Morgan also knew that a low-carb, low-fat, low-anything fad diet was simply out of the question. The 8-Hour Diet gave her the flexibility she needed to lose weight while juggling her schedule as a full-time accountant and single mom.

A SIMPLE SOLUTION—WITH SOME WIGGLE ROOM
Morgan's day starts at 5:30 a.m., when her 1-year-old son wakes up. Between her rigorous accounting job and playing Supermom, she doesn't have time to cook healthy meals for herself or the money to invest in expensive weight-loss plans. "Counting calories and carbs is not something I have time for. I looked at Weight Watchers, I looked at Atkins, I looked at a lot of different things, and all of it just seemed so time-consuming. I happened upon the 8-Hour Diet, and I thought, you know what? I can do that!"

LOSING WEIGHT THE HEALTHY WAY
The 8-Hour Diet didn't restrict Morgan's calories, so she was able to get the energy and nutrients she needed as a breastfeeding mom while still losing weight. And because she never felt constrained, it was easier to eat well. "Knowing that I could have a candy bar if I wanted helped me make healthier decisions because I didn't feel that deprivation," she says. "It really fit right in with me."

SETTING ASIDE HER SELF-DOUBTS
Morgan has dropped 15 pounds so far, and she's feeling the ripples across all areas of her life. "I've lost weight, I feel better, and making healthier choices has made me feel better about myself," she says. "That confidence carries over into everything you do—work, your social life, your personal life." She has more energy to play with her son, and her outlook has changed radically, she says, as a result of the 8-Hour Diet. "It makes me feel pretty. Beautiful. I used to wonder, am I not good enough, or pretty enough, or something like that? And losing the weight has really helped me. Just that boost of confidence makes me feel better about my life in general." Morgan has recommended the plan to friends and family and says she'll stick with it for the long term. "It was the ideal diet for me!"

where will tell you that if you just don't eat that, or if you only eat it in some sort of mystical combination with other foods, you'll be fine.

Different kind of diet, but the same result: You can try to live on steak and eggs, but eventually you need a slice of bread. And a pat of butter. In the long run, these fad diets don't work, either.

The 8-Hour Diet is different because you can eat any kind of food you want, in any quantity you want. According to researchers at the Regulatory Biology Laboratory at the Salk Institute for Biological Studies, "When we eat may be as important as what we eat." They first stumbled upon this stunning breakthrough in animal studies. When they gave mice the run of the house—let them eat whatever they wanted, but only during a set period of time—the mice lost weight. When they put mice on a restricted diet and fed them throughout the day, they gained weight. Their stunning conclusion: You can eat whatever you want because by limiting the period of time in which you're consuming food, you actually increase the number of calories—especially fat calories—your body burns during the day.

That's why the 8-Hour Diet is such a paradigm shift. This plan eliminates willpower. It eliminates sacrifice. And it eliminates calorie-counting, glycemic-index crunching, carb-fat-protein balancing, point totaling, and other Einsteinian mathnastics that have turned ordering dinner into an arithmetic problem worthy of Harvard Business School.

Instead, just eat whatever you want, as much as you want.

But only eat during an 8-hour period each day.

And you only have to follow the diet a few days a week.

In the coming chapters, I'll explain how easy this program can be. I'll shock you with research that demonstrates how dramatically you can slash your risk of diabetes, heart disease, cancer, and even degenerative brain diseases such as Alzheimer's. And I'll introduce you to eight foods you should eat every day to ensure you're getting all the nutrients your body craves. (Don't worry, you've probably already eaten most of the eight today! And there's not a rice cake in sight!)

And throughout this book, you'll meet some of the men and women whose lives have been changed by the 8-Hour Diet: People like Morgan Jennings, a single mom who dropped 15 pounds in 6 weeks, even while breastfeeding. ("It was the ideal diet for me," she says.) Or Marisa DeLorenzo, who dropped 13 pounds in 6 weeks and felt more energetic than ever. ("My pants fit better and even my face looks slimmer," she reports.) Or Billy Long, a Missouri congressman who dropped more than 3 pounds a week and wants to share his success with others: "Man, if you knew about the 8-Hour Diet, it'd change your life!" he says.

Start Losing Weight—Today!

Still skeptical? Believe me, you're not going to find anyone more skeptical of diet trends, fads, and "breakthroughs" than I am. I've spent the last 20 years of my life following—and sometimes swallowing—every new bit of nutrition and exercise science that comes my way. As a health editor, I spend my days poring over studies and news coverage of what's happening in the field of exercise and weight loss.

And I know from personal experience how hard it can be to lose that extra weight. As a latchkey kid growing up in a single-parent household, I had no one to tell me when to stop eating. My dad was gone, and my beloved mom worked day and night trying to keep food in the house. I, on the other hand, worked day and night trying to empty food from the house, noshing and nibbling from the moment I got up until the moment I passed out in front of a *Twilight Zone* rerun, with a pack of Twizzlers by my head. By the time I was 14, I had packed on more than 200 pounds. I was one lazy, lipid lad.

Then I got a cold slap of reality that changed everything. I never thought that growing up in a single-parent household struggling to afford college would be an advantage in life, but it actually was. To earn my degree, I had to join the Navy Reserve—and that's when my life changed. Gone was my 24-hour noshing cycle. You ate when the Navy told you to eat, and my mates and I would descend on the mess hall like hyenas on a wounded water buffalo. But when mess was over, it was over—no continuous snacking when you're part of a construction battalion, toppling trees and moving tons of earth to build a runway, as we were trained to do in the Seabees.

Soon I began to lose weight. I credited it to the rigors of basic training, and when I left the Navy and joined *Men's Health*, I remained an avid exerciser, even completing the New York City Marathon. But over the last few years, I've come to understand that eating the military way might well have been the breakthrough my body needed. In other words, eating as much as you want of whatever you want, but only during a set period of the day.

See, as a diet and fitness expert, I'm always on the lookout for a foolproof weight-loss plan. And usually I'm disappointed in the long-term results. Indeed, I created the *New York Times* bestselling *Eat This, Not That!* series for exactly that reason—I simply just hadn't found a diet plan that worked perfectly for everyone. *Eat This, Not That!* taught people how to lose weight without dieting—making simple swaps, still eating their favorite foods but saving hundreds of calories by choosing one brand over another. And millions of people lost 10, 20, 30—sometimes 100 pounds!—following these simple swaps.

But as successful as *Eat This, Not That!* has been, I've never seen research that can solve the one missing link of weight loss—how can we make the body burn its own fat stores preferentially? And how can we extend life span, prevent disease, and improve brain function through food? Perhaps, I thought, we never will.

Yet over the last couple of years, a new area of science has emerged, and I've been following it—closely, but

"I THINK IT'S THE PERFECT PLAN!"

Congressman Billy Long lost 20 pounds and regained control of his health—in just 6 weeks!

Billy Long, 57, SPRINGFIELD, MISSOURI

OCCUPATION: **US REPRESENTATIVE, MISSOURI'S 7TH DISTRICT**
HEIGHT: **6'1"**   STARTING WEIGHT: **315**   WEIGHT AFTER 6 WEEKS: **295**

Missouri's 7th District Representative Billy Long always had a hearty appetite, but playing basketball and football as a teenager helped him keep his weight in check. Over the years, though, his love of food caught up with him—and when he was elected to Congress, his crazy schedule and a heap of after-hours events made exercising and eating healthfully an even bigger challenge. "Evening snacking was always my problem. I'd eat Oreos, I'd eat cheese—you'd be appalled!" says Long. With the 8-Hour Diet, Rep. Long was able to drop the extra weight without resorting to prepackaged food or a tangle of rules to follow—it's exactly what he was looking for. "I think it's the perfect plan," he says.

LOSING POUNDS: "IT'S EASY!"
Representative Long has to travel and socialize for his job, so a rigid diet wasn't an option. "A lot [of diets] want you to eat four or five or six small meals throughout the day, and you're trying to stop what you're doing and eat a power bar or mix up a shake—but there's none of that with this. You go out to dinner with your family and you order the same stuff they do. It's easy!" Long could make small tweaks to his usual routine—cutting down from six pieces of bacon to two, or swapping in cottage cheese for his usual fries alongside a burger—without missing out entirely. "I've cut down my portion sizes, and I've quit eating after 8 o'clock at night—it's just a matter of retraining myself," says Long.

"IT'LL CHANGE YOUR LIFE"
A mere 6 weeks in, Long has already shed 20 pounds and seen his health and life change dramatically. "It's easier to get up out of a chair. Easier to get on and off airplanes," he says. "I'm more motivated. It's just easier to do things; you have more energy." It's an eating plan he can stick to. He's hoping to get down to 200 pounds with the help of the 8-Hour Diet and next summer to be batting in the annual Congressional Baseball Game. His success has been so motivating that he's eager to recommend the plan to others. "I see people walking through the airport all the time who are obviously, like me, carrying too much weight. And I look at 'em and I think, man, if you knew about the 8-Hour Diet, it'd change your life!"

The Least Important Meal of the Day

Let me apologize on behalf of an entire country full of fitness gurus, diet-book authors, trendy nutritionists, weight-loss clinics, unemployed actors working in gyms, and people who scream at chunky people on TV for a living. Almost all of us have been feeding you a line of bull. And we've been feeding it to you for breakfast.

I'm a big believer in science. But sometimes science gets it wrong. Like back in the early 1990s, when we were told by the US government that we could eat whatever we wanted, as long as it was "low fat." So we all chowed down on bagels, bread, pasta, and fat-free cookies. Except, that "fat-free" stuff wasn't free at all; by shocking our bodies with big doses of carbohydrates, the fat-free craze just increased our risk of obesity and diabetes.

Turns out, the same is true of the expert advice to eat a big, hearty breakfast. We've all seen the "facts": People who regularly skip breakfast are 450 percent more likely to be obese. People who go for a period without eating lose muscle, not fat. People who eat a big breakfast "jump-start" their metabolism and burn more calories.

Except it's simply not true.

Consider a study published in *Nutrition Journal* in 2011. Researchers followed the eating habits of 100 normal-weight and 280 obese participants during a 2-week period. They found that in both groups, the more calories they ate at breakfast, the more total calories they ate for the rest of the day. And when they ate a smaller breakfast, or none at all, their total calorie intake was less.

Conclusion: Overweight people should "consider the reduction of breakfast calories as a simple option" to lose weight.

In fact, more and more research is proving that avoiding calories in the morning is the way to stay not only slim, but also strong in both body and mind. In fact, this strategy can completely erase the damage of an otherwise "bad" diet.

In a 2010 study in the *Journal of Physiology*, researchers fed a group of active men an unhealthy diet composed of 50 percent fat and 30 percent more calories than they normally consumed. They then divided the men into three subgroups: one group didn't exercise at all, another group exercised four times a week after eating breakfast, and the third group exercised four times a week before eating their first meal of the day. The no-exercise group gained 6 pounds, developed insulin resistance, and began storing extra fat in their muscle cells. The group that exercised after eating breakfast gained about 3 pounds and also showed signs of insulin resistance and greater fat storage. But the participants who exercised before eating their first meal gained almost no weight and showed no signs of insulin resistance.

So why have we been lectured to about "the most important meal of the day" for all these years? "There are a lot of forces in our society pushing against" skipping breakfast, says Mark Mattson, PhD, chief of the Laboratory of Neurosciences at the National Institute on Aging, whom you'll hear more from in the pages to come. "Those forces are driven by money. They include the food industry obviously, and in some respects the pharmaceutical industry." Breakfast cereals alone are an $11 billion a year industry, and that's before you get into eggs and bacon, bagels and lox, pancakes and syrup. There are a lot of different businesses relying on your morning meal to make their budgets.

So before we all go hog wild on bacon and do the chicken dance over eggs, let's take a second look at the research. This book is going to change everything about how you view breakfast.

And the good news: Skip breakfast, and you can set your alarm clock just a few minutes later!

skeptically—ever since. And now I'm convinced. In this book, I'm going to lay out the irrefutable evidence and teach you how to change your body and your life forever.

We'll begin diving deeper in Chapter 1: I'll lay out the other salutary effects of the 8-Hour Diet and explain how this program works on a cellular level, turbocharging the mitochondria that fuel your body and rev your metabolism. Then we'll dive further into some very cool, very surprising science in Chapter 2, where we visit the Salk Institute in LaJolla, California, to talk with the foremost researchers in the field. What they're helping us to understand is that our bodies are something like clockworks, preferring to schedule maintenance and system backup during planned downtimes. You'll learn why and how weight loss becomes so rapid and so easy to accomplish.

I am a skeptic, just like you. But I'm convinced: The 8-Hour Diet is the easiest, most effective weight-loss plan ever created. And it's right here in your hands.

THE 8-HOUR DIET CHEAT SHEET

This at-a-glance guide shows how easy it is to change your body—and your life!

The 8-Hour Eating Plan

DURATION 8 hours a day, during which you can, and should, eat whenever you want

DAYS/WEEK The magic of the 8-Hour Diet is that you don't have to follow it every day. Seven days a week? Terrific! Only five? You're still good! Just three? You'll still see benefits!

MEALS As many as you want, whenever you want—as long as they fall within your 8-hour eating plan

FOODS At each meal or snack, try to get two of the eight Powerfoods, one Fat Buster, and one Health Booster. Every day you want to make sure you can say, "I ate my 8!"

THE FAT BUSTERS	THE HEALTH BOOSTERS
Turkey, eggs, and lean meats	Raspberries and other berries
Walnuts and other nuts	Oranges, apples, and other fruits
Yogurt and other dairy	Spinach and other green vegetables
Beans, peanuts, and other legumes	Whole grain breads, cereals, and oatmeal

PERFECT SNACK EXAMPLES Hummus with carrots; yogurt with blueberries; green salad with walnuts; roast beef and tomato sandwich

FOODS TO EMPHASIZE Lean protein; fiber; healthy (mono- and polyunsaturated) fats; brightly colored fruits and vegetables

FOODS TO LIMIT Refined carbohydrates such as baked goods; sugar; white bread, rice, and pasta; saturated and trans fats; high-fructose corn syrup

THE CARB RULE Always include two Powerfoods in any carb-heavy snack or meal (e.g., pasta with cheese and tomato sauce; sandwich with turkey and lettuce; cereal with milk and berries; chips with bean dip and salsa).

BEVERAGES Dramatically reduce your calorie intake by drinking more water and skipping sugary drinks. Limit alcohol to two or three drinks per week to maximize your results.

EXERCISE Optional. But 8 minutes each morning (Yes, just 8 minutes!) is enough to start turbocharging your weight loss.

SKIPPING DAYS, CHEATING, AND GENERALLY MESSING UP Totally allowed.

The Ground- breaking Science Behind the 8-Hour Diet

Discover how this revolutionary plan works—on a cellular level!

Walk into my office at *Men's Health* on any given workday (and plenty of nights and weekends), and you won't see an inch of open space on my desk. What you'll see instead are stacks of research papers, charts, and graphs, all reporting the latest findings on fitness and weight loss. The chairs will be piled high with books and DVDs sent to me by this doctor or that exercise guru, each with a new plan to strip off pounds, fight disease, and improve readers' lives. Frankly, it's a mess in here. Occasionally, when the office gets too cold, I realize I've allowed the files and folders to spill over on top of the heating vents, and I know it's time to do a little housecleaning.

In other words, my office isn't built for comfort. It's built for research. And most of the facts, figures, and findings that come my way have been variations on the same thing, year after year after year.

Until I discovered the science behind the 8-Hour Diet.

It's hard to overstate how important, how revolutionary, and how life-altering this research is. And it's hard to overstate how quickly and easily you'll begin to see results. By carving out an 8-hour window in which to eat to your heart's content, you'll burn your body's fat stores effortlessly. You'll dramatically decrease your risk of disease. And, most amazingly of all, you'll significantly slow the aging process. Add in just a bit of exercise before your first meal—an 8-minute walk around the block will do—and you turbocharge the results.

The science behind the weight-loss and antiaging benefits is simple—yet groundbreaking. And it actually operates in two ways. First, the 8-Hour Diet powers up your mitochondria—the "battery packs" in your cells that form the basis of your metabolism. Second, the 8-Hour Diet actually resets your body's calorie-burning mechanism, allowing it to burn body fat for energy. No other plan has ever fully turned the key on these two weight-loss secrets, because the science behind how they operate simply hadn't been brought to light.

Until now.

The Science of Cellular Metabolism

Within every cell in your body is a posse of organelles (or miniature organs) called mitochondria.

If you were a clerk at Home Depot, you'd have trouble figuring out exactly where in the store to shelve the mitochondria. You might, for example, stock them in the electrical supply aisle because one of their main functions is sending electrical signals through the cells; as such, they operate like millions of dimmer switches, increasing and decreasing the flow of energy through your body as needed.

Or, you might store them in the gardening section because another role of these microscopic organelles is to both promote and prune back the growth of cells. Mitochondria control cell regeneration, triggering the birth of fresh new cells even as they order older cells to self-destruct once they outgrow their preprogrammed life span. In that way, properly functioning mitochondria are critical to our staying young by keeping new cells always at the ready; but they're also critical to reducing the incidence of cancer—which is essentially caused by out-of-control cell growth.

But most likely, the store manager would tell you to shelve your mitochondria with the home generators because mitochondria are most often referred to as the power plants of the cells. They produce most of the body's supply of adenosine triphosphate (ATP), the chemical energy source that is, in its most basic role, the very stuff of life. ATP is the final end product of your salami sandwich—the energy that fuels everything from the wiggle in your fingertips to the growth of your toenails.

Now, here's the key thing you need to know about mitochondria: Like any other sort of engine, they generate energy, but they also generate waste. However, unlike your car engine, which turns gasoline into energy while creating smog, the mitochondria turn food into energy while creating something called *free radicals*.

And these free radicals aren't peaceful hippies who want to give you a bouquet of organic kale and turn you on to Phish. Free radicals are the source of almost all the ills in your body. The prime movers of the aging process, free radicals impede the function of mitochondria, killing off cells and, eventually, causing your downfall—from cardiovascular disease, cancer, diabetes, Alzheimer's, or some other age-related illness. Free radicals are oxygen molecules; fighting them is the role of those antioxidants that every juice carton and vitamin bottle in the supermarket is boasting about. But dietary antioxidants like vitamins A, C, and E, while vital for good health, can have only a limited effect on free radicals produced by our mitochondria; otherwise, given all the vitamins we pop, we'd all be living to 200 and putting those plastic surgeons on *Extreme Makeover* out of work.

So the mitochondria are the good cop *and* the bad cop. They make the ATP that keeps you alive, but in the process, they create the free radicals that lead to your demise. What's a well-meaning microscopic organelle to do?

The 8-Hour Cellular Solution

Like any engine, the mitochondria in your cells will burn fuel more efficiently, produce more energy, and throw off less waste if they are properly maintained. But our current morning-to-midnight eating schedule does the exact opposite. Humans actually evolved to eat only a few hours a day (you'll read more about this in the next chapter). When we spend too many of our hours eating, the mitochondria don't get a break from processing calories. The engines run hot, generating a

"I DIDN'T THINK I COULD LOSE WEIGHT THAT FAST!"

Andre dieted just 3 days a week—and lost 15 pounds in 6 weeks!

Andre Charles, 21, ATLANTA, GEORGIA

OCCUPATION: **STUDENT**   HEIGHT: **5'11"**

STARTING WEIGHT: **200**   WEIGHT AFTER 6 WEEKS: **185**

Late night snacks. A crazy-busy schedule. Constant stress. The daily life of a student isn't the most conducive for weight loss. But with the 8-Hour Diet, Andre Charles was able to shave off excess pounds without losing his academic edge.

A LIFETIME OF BAD HABITS—GONE!

Andre had always struggled with his weight, a problem compounded by his sedentary lifestyle. As a teen, he was more likely to be found playing video games than playing hoops. But when he tipped the scales at 240 pounds, he knew he needed a change. "I feel as though I've been eating wrong my entire life," he says. On the 8-Hour Diet, Andre added smart food choices to his grocery list, loading up on new healthy favorites such as Greek yogurt and fruit. He also kicked his greatest vice: after-hours snacking. "[At first I didn't like] not being able to eat late at night," Andre says. "But it was a habit the diet helped me out of."

8 MINUTES TO LEAN

Andre increased his activity level by incorporating some of the optional 8-Minute Workouts into his morning routine. "Once I started doing it consistently, it increased my metabolism," he says. Plus, it gave him the incentive to find more time in his schedule to devote to exercise. The result? Fifteen pounds gone in just 6 weeks, plus a slimmer waist and smaller gut. "I didn't think I could lose that much weight that quickly," he says.

A SIMPLE PLAN FOR LONG-TERM SUCCESS

Andre is not the only person who has noticed his transformation. "People say they see a difference in how I present myself," he says. "They say I seem more confident now." When he reveals the remarkably simple plan he followed to change his body and his life, "[everyone] wants to try it immediately because of my quick change," Andre explains. And the ease of the plan has become the main selling point: "There isn't one reason why you could ever fail at this," he says. "Planning meals between certain hours instead of restricting or eliminating your normal meals made it very simple to follow. I didn't have to make an extreme change to what I ate, just when I ate it."

Continued

Continued

PURSUING A BETTER BODY
Andre's rapid weight loss was so easy, he's determined to keep going.
Although he started off by following the 8-Hour Diet just 3 days a week,
Andre says he wants to continue on a daily basis in the hopes of losing even
more. "I want to cut down to 175 and build muscle on top of that," he says.
"If I follow the diet, I can make that happen."

lot of free radicals—which then damage the very mitochondria that produced them. It's like running your car day and night and never stopping to change the oil. As the mitochondria become damaged, they also lose their ability to regulate cell growth and to process food efficiently. The result: You start to age, and you start to gain weight, as the energy in your food is stored as fat instead of being turned into ATP.

The 8-Hour Diet is designed to allow the mitochondria to function at their most efficient, keeping you slimmer, younger, healthier. According to a 2009 study from Texas Tech University, when food is broken down faster than it is replaced—either by exercise or by taking a break from eating—ATP levels increase. There's also an increase in the breakdown of fatty acids and in glucose (energy) uptake, along with a decrease in the creation of fatty acids and glucose in the liver. In other words, you get more energy, more fat burn, and less fat storage. In another study, Italian researchers found that limiting the time in which you're eating protected against inflammation and oxidative damage to the heart. More efficient mitochondria equals greater fat burn, a slowing of the aging process, and protection against disease.

In fact, on the 8-Hour Diet, your body can actually increase the number of mitochondria in your cells (a process known as *mitochondrial biogenesis*); the more mitochondria you have, the less each individual organelle has to work, and the fewer free radicals are produced. "This type of eating plan not only protects the mitochondria from damage, it increases their proliferation," says Mark Mattson, PhD, chief of the Laboratory of Neurosciences at the National Institute on Aging. In a 2009 study from the Pennington Biomedical Research Center in Louisiana, subjects who followed a meal-limitation program for 6 months saw their mitochondrial DNA content increase by 35 percent! (A control group who ate whenever they wanted saw no such change.)

Imagine the effects on your health: You lose weight rapidly, and you slow the aging process. "What we're learning is that [mitochondria] play a significant role in neurodegenerative diseases and metabolic syndrome, which is a more amorphous designation that reflects an epidemic of obesity," says Michael Holsapple, PhD, vice president of the Society of Toxicology. "We see this as cutting-edge science." And, according to a paper published by the University of California-San Diego, heart cells have more mitochondria than any other body cells. So protecting your mitochondria disproportionately lowers your risk of heart disease.

But that's only part of the story behind the 8-Hour Diet. Maybe you don't care about preventing aging, stopping heart disease, or reducing your risk of cancer—you just want to look good in a swimsuit, and fast. (That's a little short-sighted, but hey, *any* motivation will do.) In that case, there's another scientific angle that you might find even more exciting: This plan completely changes the way in which your body burns body fat.

Unlocking the Body's Fat Stores

Your body stockpiles calories in two ways: as quick-burning glycogen, which is contained in the liver and muscles, and as slow-burning fat, which is stored, well, pretty much everywhere else. What makes weight loss so difficult is that your

"I'M MORE COMFORTABLE IN MY OWN SKIN!"

Laura lost 12 pounds in 6 weeks— without sacrificing her favorite foods

Laura Qualley, 28, ALLENTOWN, PENNSYLVANIA

OCCUPATION: **SUBSTITUTE TEACHER**   HEIGHT: **5'7"**
STARTING WEIGHT: **152**   WEIGHT AFTER 6 WEEKS: **140**

Laura was thrilled when she and her fiancé bought a house together, but their shared love of cooking in their new kitchen was causing her weight to creep up. She started to feel uncomfortable with her body, but she didn't want to sacrifice her social life to slim down. "I love to go out with people, and I don't want to be the person at the table saying 'Oh, I can't eat that!'" With the 8-Hour Diet, says Laura, she was able to make her weight-loss plan fit her life, and not the other way around.

SLIMMING DOWN—SANS SACRIFICE

"Clothes weren't fitting right, so I thought, if I could just slim down, then I'd feel a lot better," Laura says. But she didn't want to cut out her favorite foods. "There are just certain things that I love that I'm not willing to give up," she explains. On the 8-Hour Diet, Laura was able to keep eating favorite foods like cheesesteaks and wings by timing her meals, while tweaking her habits by adding in lean proteins, fruits, and vegetables.

SMALL CHANGES, BIG RESULTS

Laura saw results on the 8-Hour Diet almost immediately—friends and family started commenting on how good she looked within the first 2 to 3 weeks, and by the end of her third week on the plan, Laura had already dropped 8 pounds! "If you're looking to shed pounds and feel better about yourself, this is an easy change to work into your life," Laura says. "I saw the payoff in a few weeks!" Her quick losses helped motivate her, and now she's happier than ever with her body. "Twelve pounds may not be a lot for some people, but for me it was. I'm much more comfortable in my own skin. That's always been the ultimate goal—not a number on the scale, but just feeling good about how I look. And over the past few weeks, [the 8-Hour Diet] has definitely helped me reach that point."

body is programmed to hold on to that fat; tapping it for energy is hard. But it's exactly what this program will encourage your metabolism to do.

The first thing your body does when you wake up each morning is to start looking for energy to burn—hey, that snooze button isn't going to hit itself! And it goes right for that fast-and-easy glycogen in the liver. "There's about 1,500 to 2,000 calories in there," says Dr. Mattson.

But then you get up and pour a bowl of cereal, or you grab a coffee and Danish on the way to work, or maybe you skip breakfast altogether and simply start snacking around 11 or so. Regardless, your body now has a brand new source of glycogen to burn—food! And if more food comes in than your body can burn, it starts to break it down and store it—putting some of it back in your liver as glycogen, and some of it you-know-where as fat. Day after day, this goes on, until you wake up 10 years later and look nothing like your high school yearbook photo.

Now, what if you could torch all that glycogen early in the day and program your body to start burning fat instead?

That's what the 8-Hour Diet does. With the most moderate bit of exercise—a mere 8 minutes a day before your first meal—you'll begin to burn through these glycogen stores like a 13-year-old girl through a Justin Bieber fanzine and spend more of your day in fat-burning mode. (More about this in a minute.) And by not snacking late at night, you'll further deplete these glycogen stores, so that when you wake up the next day, fat burning will start even sooner. "You're switching to using fats instead of what's in your liver," says Dr. Mattson. "There's going to be a reduction in the size of your fat stores."

This technique—limiting the time period in which you eat to tap your body's fat stores—is known as "intermittent fasting." And that's what the 8-Hour Diet is all about.

8 Hours, 8 Minutes, 8 Foods

There's something appealing about the figure 8—broad at the top, solid at the bottom, lean in the middle. It's a perfect metaphor for the fit and healthy body we all aspire to.

Unfortunately, I spent most of my early life looking less like an 8 and more like a big, fat 0. You know what I'm talking about—that creeping middle spread that doctors call "apple shaped." Belly fat—the most insidious form of fat there is—increases your risk of all the major diseases of our time, from heart disease and diabetes to cancer, stroke, and even sexual dysfunction. And our open-all-night eating style creates dysfunction at the cellular level, literally confusing the mitochondria that are supposed to keep us young, healthy, and lean.

The 8-Hour Diet is designed to counteract that growing expanse around your middle and carve you back into the lean, strong, shapely 8 that screams out young, fit, and healthy. And it's designed to help you do it without spending hours in the gym, without spending hundreds of dollars on fitness classes, and without leaving a trail of sweat behind you as you jog down the road. In fact, you don't actually need to "work out" at all. You just need to get moving for 8 minutes a day, a few days a week.

Screeech! Hold up! Did the health and fitness editor just tell you not to work out? Well, not quite. I'm an enormous fan of exercise—I run and lift weights nearly every day because being in the best possible shape is part of my job. I strongly recommend you work out, too, because strenuous exercise not only boosts the effects of your weight-loss plan but also helps to beat stress and sculpt a leaner, fitter form. But if you want rapid, sustainable weight loss, you don't need to sign your paycheck over to Nike. Just 8 minutes a day, before your first meal of the day, is all you really need.

How is that possible? Doesn't it take hours on the treadmill just to burn off a Twinkie? (Actually, it would take a 155-pound man about 15 minutes of jogging to burn off a Twinkie. Which is a lot of time to spend burning off something you ate in less than a minute.)

And that's exactly why I don't want you to try to burn off calories through exercise—I want you to program your body to do that, automatically. You'll do that by depleting those glycogen stores I mentioned earlier in this chapter. Because your body doesn't have food calories to burn first thing in the morning, it's going to tap into the glycogen stores in your liver.

Here's the great news: If you did nothing but press numbers on the remote for the 16 hours you're not eating, you'd still come close to tapping all the glycogen in your liver. A 185-pound man in his late 40s would burn about 1,275 calories just sleeping or sitting still for those 16 hours; a 160-pound woman of the same age would burn about 1,073. That's your resting metabolic rate—the number of calories your body burns while at complete rest. And that's assuming you didn't do the dishes, walk the dog, take out the garbage, tuck in the kids, chase the cat off your favorite chair, climb the stairs, get undressed, hang up your clothes, roll around in bed with your partner, or do any of the physical things you would normally do after you finished eating dinner.

Now remember, there are only between 1,500 and 2,000 calories total in your glycogen stores. So by the time you wake up, you're already getting close to finishing off those stores. The 8 minutes you spend doing light exercise—even just a brisk walk around the block—before your first meal accelerates that glycogen burn, and once those stores are depleted, you'll turn into a fat-burning machine for the rest of the day.

And you'll keep burning fat, even while you eat—no matter what you eat. Meanwhile, you're further helping the mitochondria in your cells generate energy more efficiently, cutting down on your risk of disease.

Okay, a quick reality check: I know I said that you can

Graze Anatomy

Why you don't have to eat all the time to burn fat and build lean, strong muscle.

I used to work with a guy who was obsessed with building muscle. He lifted weights a lot, and he got pretty big, but the body part that got the most working out was his jaw. See, my friend bought into the well-established—but newly debunked—theory that to build and maintain lean muscle mass, you had to be constantly eating, so as to "feed your muscles." And you've probably been told, like he was, that "grazing" during the day is key to keeping your metabolism high and your body burning calories.

My friend was so obsessed with feeding his muscles that he used to come to work every day with a whole roasted chicken under his arm. He'd stick it in the office fridge, and all day long, he'd walk back and forth from his office to the kitchenette to tear off a hunk of fowl. He'd even show up in meetings with a thighbone in his paw. I was afraid we'd come to the office one morning and find a horde of cats howling outside like 13-year-old girls at a One Direction concert.

Problem is, all that eating made him a pretty large guy, and not just in the muscle department. (Also, gnawing on a chicken bone in the middle of a staff meeting is just not a great career builder, unless you're in Henry VIII's inner circle.) And more and more research has been showing that the theory of eating six times a day—three meals and three snacks—to burn fat and build muscle just doesn't hold water. In fact, your metabolism will run hotter and your muscle-making factories will work overtime when you eat less frequently. Consider:

EATING LESS FREQUENTLY HELPS YOU KEEP OFF WEIGHT. A 2010 study in the *British Journal of Nutrition* found that participants who ate three meals and three snacks per day had no greater weight loss than those who ate just three meals per day, calories being equal. "Grazing" did nothing for weight loss.

EATING LESS FREQUENTLY BOOSTS YOUR STAY-YOUNG, LEAN-MUSCLE HORMONES. Scientists at the Intermountain Medical Center in Utah asked participants to fast for 24 hours and then compared their blood samples to those taken after a

day of normal eating. They discovered that the male participants' levels of human growth hormone (HGH)—which protects
lean muscle and regulates metabolism—were 20 times higher
on the days when they fasted.

EATING LESS FREQUENTLY MAINTAINS MUSCLE FUNCTION.
A 2012 research review in the *Journal of Sports Science* found
that athletes who maintain their total energy and macronutrient
intake, training load, body composition, and sleep length and
quality are unlikely to suffer any substantial decrease in
performance during fasting for Ramadan, the Muslim religious
observance. And a 2011 study in the journal *Obesity Reviews*
found that while intermittent fasting had the same effect on
weight loss and fat loss as simply cutting calories, intermittent
fasting seemed to be more effective for retaining lean muscle
mass.

This is actually great news, because being able to eat
whatever you want, in whatever quantity you want—and not
having to make sure you've always got the right food on hand to
"stoke your metabolism"—takes a lot of pressure off. (Studies
have even shown that the more rigid your "diet" plan, the higher
your BMI was likely to be and the more depressed you were
likely to feel.)

And besides, who wants their desk to smell like a drum-
stick?

eat whatever you want, in any quantity you want. And that's true. But I'm not going to tell you that you can live on a daily regimen of nothing but Slim Jims and tequila. Yes, all of your favorite foods are allowed—from mashed potatoes to meatball heroes to Mississippi mud pies. But at the same time, your body needs enough real nutrition to go about its daily business, like breathing and digesting and making your hair grow.

To ensure you get all the nutrients your body needs—so you can go back to the mashed potatoes, meatball heroes, and mud pies—I'll introduce you to the 8-Hour Powerfoods. Foods high in protein, fiber, and healthy fats (the Fat Busters) will help your body build and maintain lean muscle, burn off flab, and fend off hunger. And foods high in vitamins and minerals (the Health Boosters) will improve your mood, ward off disease, and even help you think faster and more clearly. (I'll go into the science of these foods in Chapter 5.) Indeed, award-winning chef and food journalist Matt Goulding, my coauthor on the Eat This, Not That! series, has even created a collection of delicious recipes that incorporate the 8-Hour Powerfoods, making it that much easier to fuel your body with the nutrients it needs. See Chapter 8.

Eating one serving of each 8-Hour Powerfood every day is easy: Heck, a bowl of yogurt with some berries and cup of chili with a side salad and you're done! In fact, there won't be a day that goes by when you won't find it easy to say, "I ate my 8!"

Excited? To learn more about how the 8-Hour Diet is going to make weight loss effortless, let me take you on a field trip in the next chapter . . .

CHAPTER

2

How the 8-Hour Diet Will Change Your Body

Strip away pounds and take control of your health

The Salk Institute, in La Jolla, California, is the epicenter of a research movement that has rocked conventional weight-loss thinking to its core.

The prime mover and shaker of this research is one Satchidananda Panda, PhD, a diminutive, energetic man whose discoveries about the new science of intermittent fasting are on the cutting edge of cutting weight.

At the moment, Dr. Panda is sitting in a dark conference room, going through a research paper that's about to be published in the journal *Cell Metabolism*.

The opening slide contains a statement as revolutionary as any in the history of weight-loss science:

When we eat may be as important as what we eat.

He lingers over that for a while, to make sure it sinks in. And it does: For the last weight-obsessed century, we may have been asking the wrong questions, and therefore getting the wrong answers, about why we're so darn fat, and getting fatter. But Dr. Panda, and researchers like him, have discovered that there is a cure for obesity. And it's not what anyone expected.

The New Rules of Weight Loss

Ask the average man or woman on the street why America has such a weight problem, and you'll inevitably get answers with some combination of these factors:

★ **IT'S THE JUNK FOOD.** Too much fat, or carbs, or processed foods, or high-fructose corn syrup, or fast food, or packaged food . . . you name it, if it tastes good on your tongue, it makes your belly bigger.

★ **IT'S THE PORTIONS.** We've supersized our meals and our bodies with them. From New York City's attempts to ban biggie sodas to the pleas of many nutritionists to avoid "portion distortion," everyone is fed up to here with being fed up to here.

★ **IT'S THE INACTIVITY.** Remember how we used to play soccer, instead of Playstationing soccer? Surf on skateboards instead of surfing the Web? Ride bikes instead of riding the sofa? Of course our sedentary lifestyle is making us fat: Remember all the calories we used to burn getting up to change the channel instead of just using the remote?

And yet . . .

★   We've tried to eat healthfully, going low-fat, low-carb, sugar-free, and organic.

★   We've tried to cut our portion sizes, count calories, follow diet plans that limit our food intake to a miserly sum.

★   We've tried exercising, forking over more than $20 billion a year to gym chains that promise to burn off more than just our disposable income.

And we just keep getting larger and unhealthier.

But finally, there may be an answer—if we just start asking the right questions.

Dr. Panda is fairly glowing here in the dark as he clicks over to a pair of US maps. The one on the left shows the night sky over the continental United States. The one on the right: diabetes incidence, county by county, in the population. The charts have been adjusted to control for the greater population numbers in city areas, but still, the two are mirror images of one another.

"Where there are more lights," he says, "there is more diabetes." The more nighttime light there is, the more midnight oil that's burned, the greater the risk for the number-one health scourge of our age.

He goes on to explain what may be happening: "My hypothesis is that staying up and eating late may be the cause. In the history of human civilization—millions of years—we didn't know how to use fire. In the daytime human beings would hunt something, eat something, but in the nighttime they had to protect themselves against predators. It was only 200,000 years ago that we learned how to control fire, and only a few people could afford to use fire to stay up past sunset. But in the last 50 years, we've had light at night. And that's where we see the rise of weight problems."

His theory: The advent of artificial light has also led to an artificial extension of our feeding times. There's a natural stop sign built into our circadian rhythms, and we run through it almost every day. That throws our digestive system, and the many hormones and enzymes that manage it, off-kilter. We can't process the food we eat, and as a result it ends up where it shouldn't—around our bellies and butts.

Not convinced yet? Hang in there.

Dr. Panda continues his presentation, describing the ingenious study his laboratory devised to test his thesis in mice. They were divided into two groups: One group was given the freedom to eat anything they wanted at any time of day. The other could eat as much as they wanted, but only within an 8-hour time frame. The test study lasted for 100 days.

With this setup, Dr. Panda called upon the mouse next to his laptop. The screen flashed the image below.

Guess which mouse had the run of the house for 24 hours?

"Simply limiting food intake to 8 hours gives you all the benefits—without worrying about food intake," Dr. Panda explains.

And the revelations didn't stop there. Mice normally eat at night, a wise choice for an animal that has to dodge cats, hawks, and shrieking housewives. But when Dr. Panda further divided the mice, giving some of them a high-fat diet and others a healthy mix of carbs, protein, and fat, he discovered that those who had access to healthy food stuck to their normal eating pattern. The mice on the high-fat diet, on the other hand, tended to expand their eating time, nibbling day and night. His conclusion: "When we eat fat-rich food, we become addicted to food, almost. It is the big question in neuroscience today. If we can disconnect that addiction, we can cure it."

In other words, the longer we stretch out our eating cycle, the fatter we get. And the more fatty foods we eat, the longer we stretch out our eating cycle.

Clearly, Dr. Panda has given a lot of thought to how this mouse research will translate into the species you and I be-

"THE 8-HOUR DIET ALLOWS YOU TO INDULGE—AND LOSE WEIGHT!"

Jill dropped 10 pounds in just 4 weeks!

Jill Martin, 36, NEW YORK, NEW YORK

OCCUPATION: **FASHION/LIFESTYLE EXPERT AND TV PERSONALITY**

HEIGHT: **5'7"**   STARTING WEIGHT: **145**   WEIGHT AFTER 4 WEEKS: **135**

Jill Martin had only a few pounds to drop, but as a busy author, fashion consultant, and television correspondent—not to mention a major foodie—she wanted a program that would give her boundaries without forcing her to overhaul her whole schedule and lifestyle. Just a month in, she's 10 pounds lighter and more energetic than ever—all thanks to the 8-Hour Diet.

A 3-DAY-A-WEEK DIET? YES!

Like a lot of people who've tried dieting before, Jill was a weight-loss skeptic. "You hear '8-Hour Diet' and the idea that you can eat whatever you want and lose weight, and you're sort of like—wow! That sounds good, sign me up! But I was skeptical at first because I thought, how could you eat whatever you want and lose weight?" Still, her interest in looking and feeling better—and her love of rich, indulgent food—inspired her to give it a shot. The catch? Because of her busy schedule, Jill realized she'd only be able to follow the plan 3 days a week.

GREAT FOOD, INSTANT ENERGY

Jill didn't eat anything special on the diet, nor did she count calories. She just limited her eating time frame for 3 out of the 7 days of the week—and within a month, her life had changed. Jill's lost 10 pounds, gained a spring in her step, found a new balance—and she's feeling healthier than ever. "I wake up with more energy, and I find myself less hungry when I first wake up," Jill says. Her favorite part? Success without sacrifice. "If you're a food person and food is important to you, which it is to me, [the 8-Hour Diet] allows you to indulge, which a lot of diets don't," says Jill. "I could never be the girl at the table not eating!"

HEALTHIER—AND HAPPIER!

Jill couldn't be happier with her success, and she says the 8-Hour Diet gave her exactly what she was looking for. "I found that for my situation, and my personality, and my schedule, this works for me." The 8-Hour Diet let Jill set boundaries where she needed them, while still allowing her to live her life—and the result is its own reward. "For me, there's nothing better than feeling healthy and being at a weight where you're comfortable and happy." And with the new strategies she's learned from the 8-Hour Diet, she has the tools she needs to be comfortable and happy for life.

long to. He sees the human body as something like an office building: Most people go into the office during the day, work for 8 hours, and go home. Then, at night, the janitorial staff comes in to clean up the trash and repair the damage. The human body operates most efficiently on the same schedule; we just don't let it.

"Just like your brain needs to sleep for repair and rest, maybe your stomach and your liver also need to rest," he says. "A huge part of food isn't just nutrition; a lot of it is toxic, things our body doesn't need. And our stomach and liver have to break them up and send them out. It's a huge amount of work, and it's causing a lot of damage to our system. The stomach lining has to regenerate once a day, and that happens in the middle of the night. This is something no one thought about: Dampening of circadian rhythm and reduction of fasting time are contributing to obesity and diabetes."

As Dr. Panda proceeds through the rest of the slides, he stops again and again to point out all the negative stuff that fat mouse is dealing with: Hypertension. Dementia. Lousy cholesterol numbers. Cancer. Being a really large—and tempting—target for any cat who happens to stroll through the lab. It's hard not to feel sorry for that rotund rodent.

Now, if this were just a mouse study, we'd have to classify it as simply interesting and move on. But that's not what the people who work at the Salk Institute are doing. Based on what they've been seeing, a lot of people in the lab have begun further experimenting—on themselves.

"In our lab, because most of the people are seeing this on a daily basis, it influences us," he says. "So it's changing behavior for almost all of us. We don't eat after 8 o'clock at night. The guy who first did this experiment, almost no member of his family has lived beyond 55. All died of obesity, diabetes, heart attack. After he saw these results, he'd eat brunch at 11 and eat dinner at 7."

Which brings us to another skinny, fit colleague of Dr. Panda's at the Salk Institute: Ron Evans, PhD, one of the world's foremost experts on biorhythms and how they affect the body. Dr. Evans is 63 years old now, but his trim form and effervescent energy speak more to an enthusiastic teenager—albeit one with gray hair and a PhD. One look at him and you begin to wonder what's in the water on this elegant seaside campus. But of course, it isn't the water they drink, it's the 8-hour diet they follow.

"I'm in better shape than I've ever been in," says Dr. Evans. "We work on this stuff and I'm convinced by what we see, what it does. Certain kinds of changes can have a big impact on your body."

Research so compelling that the foremost weight-loss doctors in the world have changed their lifestyles in response? Sounds like something worth sitting up and taking notice of. And it's not just Dr. Panda's lab that's producing these studies. Over the next two chapters, I'm going to walk you through some of the stunning new science coming out every day and show you how everything you thought you knew about eating to lose weight was wrong! I'll explain why eating whatever you want—but focusing on getting eight Superfoods into your diet, and eating them all within an 8-hour period— will change your life forever.

You see, for years we've been told, "You are what you eat." But at least we now know there's more to that nostrum. We are what we eat, sure, but we are *when* we eat, too.

8 Hours to a Leaner You

What Drs. Panda and Evans and their voluptuous vermin are discovering isn't entirely new. For the last several years, researchers have been producing remarkable weight-loss results in people as well, using this technique they call "intermittent fasting."

Don't let the f-word scare you. In this case, fasting isn't

The 8-Hour Diet Success Story

"I LOOK BETTER! I FEEL BETTER!"

Marisa lost 13 pounds in 6 weeks—and regained her body confidence

Marisa DeLorenzo, 45, BALTIMORE, MARYLAND

OCCUPATION: **PROJECT MANAGER**   HEIGHT: **5'4"**

STARTING WEIGHT: **225**   WEIGHT AFTER 6 WEEKS: **212**

Starting a new diet is easy. Sticking to it is the hard part, as Marisa DeLorenzo can tell you. Since becoming a mom, Marisa noticed her weight sneaking up, but traditional diet plans just didn't fit into her life. "I was always looking for something that I could stick to that would keep me motivated," she says. But most of the plans she encountered were either too complicated or too time-consuming. Then Marisa discovered the 8-Hour Diet.

A DIET THAT ADJUSTS TO HER DAY

Armed with the sample meal times and 8-Hour Powerfoods, Marisa quickly established a routine that worked perfectly for her—one that was so manageable she found she could consistently stick to it 7 days a week. She broke her 8 hours—from 12 p.m. to 8 p.m.—into 4 small meals per day, eating at approximately 2- to 3-hour increments. "It's easy to incorporate into your life: You just need to get into the routine of adjusting when to start eating based on your day's activities," she says. "It seemed so natural, I wondered, 'Why didn't I think of doing this before?'"

RAPID, SUSTAINED WEIGHT LOSS

Since she started the 8-Hour Diet, Marisa experienced a rapid change not just in her weight, but in her entire body. "I was consistently losing 2 pounds every week," she says. She finds it easier to wake up in the morning, and she has more energy throughout the day. "I am more productive both at home and at work. Plus, I have the motivation to exercise," she says. "I can see progress in losing weight—my waist is smaller, my pants fit better, and even my face looks slimmer," she says. "And doing something good for myself has made me happier in general."

A NEW BODY, A NEW LIFE!

Now, although Marisa may have lost weight with the 8-Hour Diet, she's gained something else: confidence. That confidence has encouraged her to participate in activities she never would have thought of trying before. Her daughter, a cross-country runner, even convinced her to pick up the sport. "Once you start to feel better, you're inspired to do other things," she says. "And you'll see more results when you want them."

about denying yourself anything. Instead, it's simply about eating whatever you want, but staying within a sensible 8-hour window. (And remember, you don't even need to do this every day. Throughout this book, you'll meet people who saw incredible results following this plan just 3 days a week.)

Fact is, you're already fasting on a daily basis. Think, for a moment, about the word *breakfast*. It is exactly the sum of its parts—the point of the day at which you break the fast you started whenever you stopped eating the night before. In the simplest terms, the 8-Hour Diet is a way of extending the period between your last snack and your "break fast," giving your body the chance to burn away your fat stores for the energy it needs.

And burn it does. Consider a study cited in the *American Journal of Clinical Nutrition* in 2007. Researchers broke their subjects into two separate groups and fed each group the same number of calories—enough for them to maintain their weight. The only difference: One group ate all their calories in three meals, spread throughout the day. The other practiced intermittent fasting, eating the same number of calories but in a restricted time frame. Among the results: Subjects who ate in a smaller window of time had "a significant modification of body composition, including reductions in fat mass."

Part of that fat burn comes simply from the body's searching around for energy and finding it in your belly. But part of it also comes from a surprising source: According to Dr. Panda's research, restricting the time period during which you eat causes your body to burn more calories throughout the day. That's right: The longer you draw out your feeding period, the lazier your body's metabolism gets. But fit your food intake into an 8-hour window, and your body steps up to the plate, burning more calories day and night!

8 Hours to a Healthier You

The folks at the Salk Institute may look lean, but it's not vanity that's driving their research team to follow an 8-hour diet. It's the importance they place on good health. In that same *American Journal of Clinical Nutrition* article, researchers asserted that if, instead of counting calories or cutting out "bad" foods, we simply trim back the period of time in which we eat, the health benefits might begin to pile up. Consider the list of conclusions the study authors found:

★ "Lower diabetes incidence and lower fasting glucose and insulin concentrations"

★ "Lower total cholesterol and triacylglycerol concentrations, a lower heart rate, improved cardiac response . . . and lower blood pressure"

★ "Decreases in lymphoma incidence, longer survival after tumor inoculation, and lower rates of proliferation of several cell types"

In other words, eating in this manner not only helps your body burn its own fat at a more prolific rate, but it also seems to be a magic bullet that protects against the three great diseases of our day: diabetes, heart disease, and cancer. Let's take a closer look at each.

How the 8-Hour Diet Beats Diabetes

Remember that map Dr. Panda had, showing diabetes incidence across the country? It might as well be a map of the zombie apocalypse, with all the lit-up dots representing where the undead flesh eaters lurk. You should do anything possible to avoid finding yourself in the middle of one of those hot spots. Diabetes may well be our nastiest national

(continued on page 30)

Sleep Your Way Younger, Slimmer, and Healthier

The magic of midnight mitochondria management

You may not know your exact cholesterol levels right now, and unless you're hooked up to a monitor, you don't know your blood pressure or your heart rate either. You can't measure your blood sugar levels without a test or your body mass index without a sophisticated scale or your hormone levels without the help of a doctor. But there is one vital sign that gives a great indication of how healthy you are, and you and you alone can measure it.

How much sleep did you get last night?

In the previous chapter, I wrote about the role of mitochondria, the battery packs in your cells that power every aspect of your life—in fact, I'll go so far as to say that mitochondrial function *is* life. Protect these cellular organelles and you live longer, leaner, and healthier. Eating right, exercising, and avoiding toxins such as cigarette smoke are three critical ways to protect mitochondria, but the fourth pillar of staying young and lean is the one that ought to be the easiest but is often the hardest: sleeping enough.

Here's why: When night falls and darkness creeps up on us, our bodies produce the hormone melatonin, a powerful sleep inducer that also acts as an antioxidant, protecting the mitochondria and helping them to function better. Melatonin has been shown to reduce the oxidative stress that's linked to Alzheimer's, Parkinson's, and Huntington's diseases, among others. A 2007 University of Texas study review concluded that not only does melatonin detoxify harmful cancer-causing free radicals, but in doing so it may also boost the effectiveness of vitamin C, another antioxidant. Melatonin also improves the mitochondria's production of ATP, the energy chemical that fuels our lives. All that repair work that goes on when you sleep. Much of it is linked to melatonin.

Sleep Your Way Younger, Slimmer, and Healthier

Continued

Now, what happens when your body senses it's time for bed, but you respond to a yawn by turning on the lights, cranking up the tube, and maybe having a cup of joe to keep you powering through the night? Hormones go haywire. Melatonin is stifled, while your body makes more of the appetite-revving chemical ghrelin and lowers its output of leptin, the hormone that tells you you're full. A study in the *Annals of Internal Medicine* found that sleep-deprived people on low-cal diets lost 55 percent less body fat than those who were well rested—and when they did lose weight, it tended to be lean muscle mass, not fat. And in a 2007 Canadian study, people who slept only 5 or 6 hours a night increased their likelihood of being overweight by 69 percent, compared with those who habitually got 7 or 8 hours. Sleep is also critical to supporting immune function (people who sleep less than 7 hours a night are three times more likely to catch cold, according to one study) and critical thinking—as anyone who's ever flunked a test after an all-nighter can attest.

So what's it going to be: Go through life Sleepy, Dopey, Grouchy, and Sneezy (not to mention Chubby)? Or more like a live wire—lean, strong, pulsing with energy? If the latter appeals to you, here are seven ways to master your mitochondria through sleep:

➤ **BE A REGULAR.** Go to sleep and wake up at the same time every day, even on weekends. A regular routine keeps your biological clock steady so you rest better.

➤ **EXERCISE, BUT NOT TOO LATE.** One thing I really like about the 8-Minute Workouts on page 210 is that you can do them so quickly that they won't interfere with your day. Exercise improves both the length and the quality of your sleep. That said, 30 minutes of vigorous aerobic exercise keeps your body temperature elevated for 4 hours, which can inhibit sleep if you do it too late.

➤ **CUT CAFFEINE AFTER 2 PM** Caffeine stays in your system for up to 8 hours, so a cappuccino, even after an early dinner, can still be messing with your mighty mitochondria at midnight.

➤ **WRITE DOWN TOMORROW'S PLAN.** Before you begin your bedtime ritual, check tomorrow's schedule. Make a list of the things you need to get done that day using some fancy new app on your smartphone. Your goal is to short-circuit those worries that pop up just as you're dozing off.

➤ **GO TO BED 20 MINUTES BEFORE YOUR BEDTIME.** Unless you can pull some sort of Houdini voodoo on yourself, falling asleep instantly isn't really an option. If you want to be asleep by 11, be in bed by 10:40 with a good book.

➤ **COOL IT DOWN.** Experts generally recommend setting your bedroom thermostat between 65 and 75 degrees, but it's really about what makes you most comfortable. The bedroom should be just a touch cooler than elsewhere in your house because the process of your body cooling induces sleep, which is why you might want to . . .

➤ **TAKE A HOT BATH BEFORE BED.** A warm bath or shower will raise your body temperature. Then, when you get out, your body will begin to cool, making you more likely to fall asleep.

plague, one that can simultaneously increase your risk for heart disease, stroke, hypertension, sexual dysfunction, blindness, limb amputations, and kidney disease.

Yes, it's that bad.

Diabetes, in a chocolate-covered nutshell, is a malfunction in the way your body manufactures insulin, a hormone that regulates energy stores. It works like this: Your digestive system turns the food you eat into glucose—the form of sugar your body uses for energy—and sends it into the bloodstream. When the glucose shows up, your pancreas releases insulin to shepherd the glucose into your cells, which powers all their functions.

That's all well and good, until you eat too many high-energy foods and produce too much glucose and too much insulin. After years of overworking the system, your body eventually begins to lose the ability to react properly to the insulin—a condition known as insulin resistance. Suddenly you have "high blood sugar," which is death to the small capillaries in your eyes, toes, and private parts. One or all of them may fail.

The 8-Hour Diet can help prevent this risk.

In a study at the University of Copenhagen, researchers found that when men fasted every other day over a 2-week period, the insulin in their bodies became more efficient at managing blood sugar. And, in a study at the National Institute on Aging, researchers compared two sets of people—one group that followed a calorie-restricted diet and a second that ate as much as they wanted, but fasted every other day. They found that "intermittent fasting resulted in beneficial effects that met or exceeded those of caloric restriction including serum glucose and insulin levels."

Benjamin Horne, PhD, at the Intermountain Medical Center Heart Institute at the University of Utah, has also studied people who stretch out the time period between meals. His conclusion: "We found something we did not anticipate, which was that people who fast also have a lower risk of diabetes. We looked at just regular diabetes, but we also looked at body mass index, baseline glucose, and fasting glucose

"THE BEST PART IS THAT IT'S SO EASY!"

Norm Schulman lost 13 pounds in 6 weeks—without exercise or cutting calories

Norm Schulman, 57, PRINCETON, NEW JERSEY

HEIGHT: **5'8"**   OCCUPATION: **ACCOUNTANT**
STARTING WEIGHT: **191**   WEIGHT AFTER 6 WEEKS: **178**

Norm Schulman had tried everything, but he was fed up with sticking to impractical restrictions—so the 8-Hour Diet was a dream come true. "This is a stroke of genius! It seems so simple, yet the concept is clearly very achievable." He opted not to do the 8-Minute Workout or stick to the eight Powerfoods—and he still lost 13 pounds in just 6 weeks, simply by switching up the timing of his usual meals.

GO AHEAD, HAVE THE MILK SHAKE!

Name a diet, and Norm had tried it before. His main problem? Norm's business life is pretty hectic—he was named New York Enterprise Report's 2012 Accountant of the Year—so restricted eating just wasn't realistic. "You go on a diet, you have to eat certain kinds of food, and you have to be cognizant of that all day," Schulman explains. "If you go out to lunch with somebody, you get water, a salad, and you've got to make sure there's no croutons, no dressing." With the 8-Hour Diet, Norm finally found a plan that fit into his life. "Instead of telling me I can't have a shake, I can have a milk shake, it's just a matter of when I have it," he says. "The best part is that it was so easy. It was more like a game than a diet, and once I got into the routine of it, there was no turning back."

"THIS IS NOT LIKE ANYTHING ELSE!"

After 6 weeks, Norm has already lost 13 pounds on the diet—and in his first week, he was already noticing changes. "My pants were looser, my shirts fit a little better." For Schulman, the feeling of all-around good health was its own reward. "I have more energy. When you lose even 12 or 13 pounds, you feel better. You feel less bloated. You feel less tired in the afternoon." Norm's success took him by surprise, and he's unhesitating in his recommendation of the plan. "Unlike other diets that put you on a regimented food program, this is strictly timing. If you've tried everything else, this is not like anything else. It's a completely different concept. If you've tried everything else, try this."

and found that people who have been routinely fasting over the years have a significantly lower body mass and blood sugar."

How the 8-Hour Diet Beats Heart Disease

Imagine eating all you want, whatever you want, and slashing your heart attack risk just by watching the clock. That was the promise offered up by a study that was delivered at the 2011 conference of American College of Cardiology. It found that people who followed a regular fasting plan— simply stretching out the period between their last meal today and their first meal tomorrow—enjoyed a 58 percent lower risk of coronary disease, compared to those who didn't follow this plan. This backed up the findings of a 2008 study of nearly 500 people, who demonstrated a similar ability to sidestep the cardiac ward with the same eating strategy.

Dr. Horne, who conducted the University of Utah study, told the *New York Times:* "[This] was not a chance finding. We were able to replicate the findings and show that people who fast routinely have a lower prevalence of coronary disease."

And do you remember the fat mouse vs. skinny mouse paradigm presented by Dr. Panda earlier in this chapter? The bloodborne markers for heart disease—inflammation, high cholesterol—were much higher in the round-the-clock rodents than they were in the 8-hour wonder mice.

Two other researchers we spoke to for this book—Krista Varaday, PhD, and Marc Hellerstein, MD—published a review of human and animal studies related to fasting in the *American Journal of Clinical Nutrition* and made the following statement in the introduction: "In terms of cardiovascular disease risk, animal alternate-day fasting data show lower total cholesterol and triacylglycerol concentrations, a lower heart rate, improved cardiac response to myocardial infarction, and lower blood pressure." Further down in the study, they reported on men and women who were put on an alternate-day fast for 3 weeks: The women saw their HDL (good) cholesterol rise, and the men saw their triglycerides (the really bad stuff) fall.

Dr. Varaday was quoted in Britain's *Daily Mail* on all of the above: "After 8 weeks of alternate-day fasting, we saw that bad cholesterol was down, along with reductions in triglycerides, blood pressure, and heart rates. And since these are all key risk indicators of heart disease, it may not only help people lose weight but also help them decrease their risk of coronary events."

How the 8-Hour Diet Beats Cancer

Cancer. Even typing the word causes a chill. There are few of us indeed who haven't had loved ones touched by the disease. Cancer happens when cells in the body, which form and divide constantly, begin to grow out of control, impeding normal bodily functions. Each moment of cell division, something that happens tens of thousands of times a day, is an opportunity for something to go haywire. But what if you could slow down that cell growth?

There are many reasons why cancer strikes, and many of them aren't fully understood. But one contributing factor to our cancer risk is our diet—specifically, the tremendous amount of food we're regularly exposing our bodies to.

The process of cell reproduction in the body is sort of like an oven—the more fuel you toss onto it, the hotter it will burn. So when we eat morning, noon, and night, we're constantly feeding that fire. But if we simply enjoy all our favorite foods in whatever quantity we want—but allow the fire to dampen for a few more hours during the day—we'll dramatically decrease our risk of cells growing out of control.

"The body is an incredibly efficient piece of equipment," says Dr. Hellerstein. "Over millions of years it's been honed to expend less energy when the fuel supply drops off." In a fasting state, cells, including cancer cells, will multiply at a greatly reduced rate.

"It prevents cancer, we think, by slowing the rate at which

all cells in the body divide," he says. "It turns the gear down—instead of your liver cells, your breast cells, your prostate cells dividing every 3 days, they divide every 6 days. The consequence is that cells don't have such a chance of becoming carcinogenic."

So let's review: By eating whatever foods you want, in whatever quantity you want, but simply limiting your food intake to an 8-hour period each day (or even every other day!), you can drop pounds rapidly and permanently, while reducing your risk of the three biggest killers in America.

It sounds like following the 8-Hour Diet is a pretty smart move. But wait, there's more. In the next chapter, I'll explain how the 8-Hour Diet really is a smart move . . . one that will actually make you smarter!

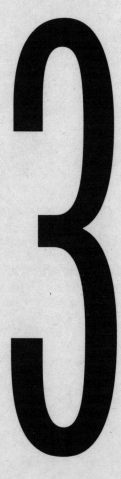

CHAPTER

3

THE 8-HOUR DIET

Longer Life, Stronger Mind

Conquer the diseases of aging and build a brain that will think better today—and tomorrow

It's Thanksgiving night. Football flickers on the flatscreen. Piles of dishes soak in a bisque-like liquid in the sink. The denuded carcass of a once-proud fowl rests in imploded squalor on the dining room table. And sprawled across assorted sofas and chairs is your family, strewn about the living room like plane crash survivors in a stuffing-induced stupor. As you survey the damage and contemplate the task of wrapping the leftovers, you feel about as energetic as a tortoise on Benadryl.

What's happening here? Why are we so lethargic after a big meal? And more important, why won't anyone help you clean up?

Contrast that scene of Turkey Day torpor with a scenario

that Professor Ron Evans from the Salk Institute conjures out on the primordial plains of Africa, where all the animals are on high alert and looking for dinner. Like Cassius in Shakespeare's *Julius Caesar*, they have "that lean and hungry look." Here's how Dr. Evans characterizes those animals that have been searching for dinner for a while: "They're aroused, always moving and alert, looking for where the food is. When they see potential prey, they're even more attentive."

Indeed, research shows that when you extend the period of time between meals—eating whatever you want in your allotted 8-hour time frame, but allowing your body the benefits of resting longer between your last meal of the day and your first meal of the next—the benefits go beyond the mere physical. (And those physical benefits—rapid weight loss, slashed diabetes risk, dramatically lowered chance of heart attack—are nothing to sneeze at.) In fact, the 8-Hour Diet may make you sharper, smarter, and calmer in the short term and make your brain healthier as you get older.

"A lot of people like to fast because they're alert and motivated," says Dr. Evans, himself an alert, motivated, intermittent faster. "That's because we're predators. When you fast, you're more attentive. Your senses of smell and sight are enhanced. Everything is heightened; your breathing, your vision, your coordination. In attack mode, animals need to be physically running so they can do the job. We do that, too. We're good at that."

So now let's become alert and attentive to one of the most profound ways that this plan can improve your life: sharpening, and extending the warranty on, your mind.

Eat Smarter, Think Smarter

It's not easy to find the fountain of youth, even if you have GPS.

If there's a secret key to unlocking eternal vigor, it's located in the laboratories of the National Institute on Aging, a short drive from downtown Baltimore. But the main drag to the research campus is under heavy renovation, so drivers lurch and bump down the strip, avoiding a pothole here and a leviathan earth-moving machine there, following detours nobody bothered to tell the folks at Garmin about, and watching flag wavers on every corner, flailing in contradictory directions.

It is, in other words, a terrific metaphor for the path that all of us are on. The road to a ripe and healthy old age is indeed populated by giant, machine-like entities, confused flag wavers, and detours that are as likely to lead to a ditch as they are to golden years that are truly gold.

But if you can read the signposts, you can find your way. In fact, there is a small one bearing the institute's initials—NIA—and it leads around the corner and down the hill to a tower so tall and so new that it is in itself a metaphor of the most promising kind. It's an emblem of the way that the best researchers, when given the best tools (thanks to the National Institutes of Health), can make progress with mysteries that have been bedeviling us since the dawn of human consciousness: Why are we destined to die, and how can we postpone that destiny for as long as possible?

If you're looking for answers—or simply looking for a way to shed weight and add energy, mental acuity, and years—there's no one better to turn to than Mark Mattson, PhD. He's been working his entire career to find ways to extend your lease—and his own—on this planet. And his solution is shockingly simple, inexpensive, and effective.

When he's not logging hours as a researcher at the National Institute on Aging, Dr. Mattson is a professor in the department of neuroscience at Johns Hopkins University School of Medicine. At a particularly brainy institution, he's in the brain department. Lately, he's been investigating the fascinating effects of caloric restriction and intermittent fasting on animals of all kinds. So, while rats and worms and rhesus monkeys command a lot of his attention, he's studying those animals for what their experiences can tell him about you and me.

"My interest in fasting began when I got interested in aging, back in the late '80s and early '90s," says Dr. Mattson, seated in his office on a high floor of the skyscraper. "It was known that in animals, if you reduce their energy intake, they live longer."

Thus began a career quest to investigate the science behind this equation: Less energy intake equals more life output. Dr. Mattson is striving to find comfortable ways to subtract food with the goal of adding productive years to human lives, including his own.

He's now in his early fifties, but he cuts the figure of a skinny teenager who just might have some difficulty keeping those blue jeans hitched above his waist. A profile in *US News and World Report* pegged Dr. Mattson's weight at "less than 130 pounds"—the result of a diet in which he skips breakfast every day, lunch most days, and relies on his evening meal for most of his sustenance.

Don't panic: Nobody's telling you to arrange your life around a single meal. But it's at least instructive that Dr. Mattson, given all he knows about this subject, has embraced this approach to eating with such fervor. Much like the researchers at the Salk Institute, the more scientists learn about the effects of an 8-hour diet, the more they begin to change their lives to gather up all its benefits.

OK, perhaps Dr. Mattson takes it to an extreme you'd rather not share. For instance, even on days he's fasting, he's known to run 6 to 9 miles with a high school cross-country team he coaches. (He says he likes to swap out snacking in favor of exercise, which isn't a bad strategy, actually.) The fact is, we could all stand to be a lot leaner and have the stamina to keep up with the teenagers in our lives. And as Dr. Mattson quickly points out, there are mental benefits as well. This distinguished doc makes his living by finding longevity secrets at a time of life when most of us would be satisfied just to locate the car keys.

So it's instructive that he calls the modern meal plan of three squares "abnormal from a genetic standpoint. We clearly haven't adapted to it yet." And by "adapted," he means that we've instead become sedentary, obese, prone to health risks, and at the mercy of fast-food advertising. Sounds like a recipe for extinction.

Dr. Mattson pulls out a fascinating set of maps that show the distances our species (or its ancestors) have traveled to find dinner over the course of our histories on the planet. The first map, from 5 million years ago, shows a dog-eat-dinosaur world where the species are constantly on the run, but cover only a limited distance. To survive long enough to reproduce, they've got to both outsmart and outrun all of the other critters that would like to eat them (or us) for dinner. Physical capacities and mental ones interlock; the species that have the best brains and endurance live the longest, have more offspring, spread their genes far and wide, and come to dominate the herd.

OK, fast forward to 10,000 years ago. A plucky mammal called homo sapiens is up on two legs and can sprint across the landscape for long distances—far outrunning even the most dogged competitor or pursuer. And for our species, this form of travel is broadening. The brains of these running animals expand because there's so much to think about: where that big bear keeps his den, where the berries ripened last spring, where the water lasted longest during the summer drought. Their muscles grow and their bellies shrink in like measure, to make it easy for them to run to those places.

So you see how the combination of a lean belly and a big brain could increase the odds that you survived a long time and mated successfully. Who wouldn't want to get busy with an animal like that?

And that's just what the 8-Hour Diet can give you.

Dr. Mattson points at his map, studded with hazards and opportunities and showing an animal that can range far and wide to guarantee his survival. Skipping meals inspires the animal to peak efficiency, physically and mentally. That's the world our bodies are genetically wired to thrive in. All of these marvelous mechanisms kick in to protect us from harm and increase our odds of thriving in a difficult environment when we trigger them with intermittent fasting.

The only bad news: We're not living 10,000 years ago. We don't need to remember where the wildebeests feed or the crocodiles roam. Today, we need only remember how many paces there are between our cubicle and the vending machine.

On to Dr. Mattson's last map, labeled, ominously, "Transition to the Sedentary/Overfed/Obese Phenotype." This Google map of gluttony shows beings who are capable of traveling much farther distances, but it strips away the hazards and hunger and replaces them with Hardees and Five Guys. In place of healthy running figures, it swaps in a little jeep symbol, which stands for "effort-sparing technologies." Plentiful food and little effort. You can probably guess what happens to the lean, healthy homo sapiens.

In the upper left-hand corner of the map, Dr. Mattson has included a damning stat. The two previous maps featured animals that had a body mass index—a measure of fat—in the 19 to 24 range, enough to sustain us if a food shortage threatens, but not undermine our health in the long run. In the current age, that BMI figure balloons above 25 and threatens everything we hold dear: our looks, our sex lives, our health, our life expectancy.

And that's why Dr. Mattson, one of the foremost anti-aging experts in the world, lives the kind of life he, and we, are genetically evolved to excel in. Here's how he pulls it off: "The fast I'm doing: Skip breakfast and lunch and exercise instead, then eat a nice meal over dinner."

Of course, Dr. Mattson gets paid to be his own guinea pig, and his is not a lifestyle that everyone would want to follow. But you don't need to be anywhere near as rigorous to see the benefits of the 8-Hour Diet. He mentions two studies he did with groups of 21st century homo sapiens, intermittently restricting meals. One study was half a year in duration, another 2 months. "The only subjects who dropped out dropped out within the first 2 weeks," Dr. Mattson says. "After 2 to 3 weeks they got to like the diet mainly because they started losing weight and started feeling better.

"It doesn't matter which fast a person does," he continues. "If they can do it and stick to it, they're going to lose weight and their health is going to improve. I think the more healthy diets that are available to people, the more likely they are to incorporate one of them into their lifestyle."

Reassuringly, it's not as if he wants you to outlive your reasons for living: "What we want to do is understand how we can help people live long lives without disease," he notes. "Have less focus on extending maximum life span—not necessarily helping people live to 150."

A Life of Living at Peak Power

If you had to name your worst nightmare about aging, what would it be—aside from still wearing leather pants at age 63, like Gene Simmons of the once-popular group Kiss?

Right: It's that you'll descend into the mental fog of Alzheimer's disease, slowly losing your cognitive powers, not recognizing your own spouse, your children, or your fellow aging ex-band members from the once-popular group Kiss.

Dr. Mattson shares that fear (except for the leather pants part). In fact, it's why he got into anti-aging research in the first place. As a neuroscientist, he's spent his entire career tracking the brain insults that lead to Alzheimer's and Parkinson's, which impair memory and movement in older people.

"One study had shown that that [intermittent fasting] will increase the life span of animals by about 30 percent," he says. The lightbulb lit up: Fasting obviously had a salutary effect on the body, but what good was a healthy body without a healthy mind? Perhaps our brains are adapted the same way our bodies are—to last longer when we take in fewer calories.

So the NIA tested a group of laboratory mice, allowing half to eat all they wanted whenever they wanted, while the other half was fed only every other day. After 3 months, the researchers administered a neurotoxin to their mousey brains. The results were definitive: The fasting mice fended off the toxins and maintained brain function; the big feeders lost their minds.

What does this mean to you, exactly?

Well, in place of the neurotoxins Dr. Mattson administered to these mice, swap in the toxic amyloids now known to cause Alzheimer's. When you fast, you increase production of proteins called *neurotropic factors* that are critical to learning and memory. They fend off brain attackers and clear the wreckage of dying cell structures, and they encourage the formation of new neurons and synapses.

To explain just how your brain grows stronger on the 8-Hour Diet, Dr. Mattson likens it to what happens to muscles when you work them regularly.

"Vigorous exercise is a stress on your muscle cells," he points out. "There's increased energy demand and increased free radicals, but it turns out to be good for your muscle cells as long as you're allowed some recovery. That mild stress stimulates muscle cells to increase production of proteins that help the cells resist stress: antioxidant enzymes, protein chaperones, growth factors, increased mitochondrial production. The number of mitochondria increase. So there's an increased ability to provide energy to the muscles."

Then he winds up to deliver the kicker: "Many of the same exact changes that are happening in the muscle cells—increased antioxidant enzymes, increased protein chaperones, increased growth factors, increased number of mitochondria—are occurring in nerve cells with fasting."

In other words, skipping meals is like exercise for your brain.

The Full-Body Fasting Effect

Dr. Mattson is talking about mental vigor here, but a study published in *Medical Hypotheses*, in 2006, extends the blanket endorsement of fasting to a whole range of debilitating conditions that can sap the life, and the joy of living, out of older people.

The study authors, Stanford-trained surgeons, write: "Since May 2003 we have experimented with alternate-day calorie restriction, one day consuming 20 to 50 percent of estimated daily caloric requirement and the next day ad lib eating, and have observed health benefits starting in as little as 2 weeks, in insulin resistance, asthma, seasonal allergies, infectious diseases of viral, bacterial, and fungal origin (viral URI, recurrent bacterial tonsillitis, chronic sinusitis, periodontal disease), autoimmune disorder (rheumatoid arthritis), osteoarthritis, symptoms due to CNS inflammatory lesions (Tourette's, Meniere's), cardiac arrhythmias (PVCs, atrial fibrillation), menopause-related hot flashes. We hypothesize that many other conditions would be delayed, prevented, or improved, including Alzheimer's, Parkinson's, multiple sclerosis, brain injury due to thrombotic stroke atherosclerosis, NIDDM [noninsulin-dependent diabetes mellitus], congestive heart failure."

The method they mention is alternate-day fasting, but as we've seen, it matters less whether you do it every day, every other day, or as little as 3 days a week. You'll still help protect yourself from all the bad things that can drain your retirement savings and ruin your golden years.

But what, exactly, is behind this "live longer, live better" effect? Dr. Mattson has one very specific, very powerful idea: Intermittent fasting improves your body's ability to clean up after itself, on a cellular level.

Think about it: You're not just a solid mass; you're a collection of individual cells carrying out very specific functions—dividing, processing nutrients, creating energy. All of that activity creates waste, in the form of free radicals—the office clutter of the human metabolism. Project that over a lifetime, where the creation of clutter outpaces its cleanup, and suddenly you can't remember the name of the guy who's been tuning up your car for three decades. You sprint to catch the bus just like you used to, but now the bus always wins.

That's aging in a nutshell: Cells have been working so hard for so long that they lose the ability to purge their waste and broken parts, and their function is compromised.

But not on the 8-Hour Diet.

When your cells are subjected to the minor stress of intermittent fasting, they can operate at peak efficiency. They do a better job of clearing out damaged cell structures and spent mitochondria, the equivalent of decommissioning the nuclear power plant before it destroys the groundwater. Less mess on the factory floor, better output from the machinery, longer operating life span for the factory, better product: you.

Live Long and Prosper

Scientists like Dr. Mattson have become convinced that intermittent fasting is an effective buffer against the major causes of death most of us have to worry about: heart disease, cancer, diabetes. Dodging or delaying those threats is in itself a profound life extender.

Says Dr. Mattson: "Dietary energy restriction can reduce tumor growth, it can protect neurons in models of neurodegenerative disorders, it can improve cardiovascular health—effects on blood pressure, for example—so being able to better understand how those changes are occurring may help us optimize those anti-aging effects."

A definitive summation of Dr. Mattson's research area appeared in *Ageing Research Reviews,* under the title "Caloric restriction and intermittent fasting: two potential diets for successful brain aging."

OK, beach reading it isn't.

But it just might be the kind of reading that could land you at the beach resort of your choosing, at age 87, still wheeling and dealing at the top of your game. For buried deep in Mattson's report is this prime nugget of science speak: "Overall, from many experimental studies . . . [intermittent fasting] seem[s] to chronically reduce the circulating levels of insulin resulting in an eventual enhanced glucose mobilization and an enhanced insulin sensitivity, both of which serve to maintain a supply of glucose for the vital organs, central nervous system, and gonads to support these critical organs in time of limited energy intake."

I'll spare you the chore of pasting that into Google Translate.

Dr. Mattson is saying that intermittent fasting (IF) torches your body's energy supplies (so bye-bye belly fat) and makes sure that every last bit of insulin is accounted for in your cells, so that your vital organs (heart, brain), central nervous system (everything attached to your brain) and gonads (yes, well . . .) are being fueled properly. Basically, your body just doesn't feel like it has the luxury of becoming fat and diabetic.

So what does that have to do with your mental acuity? And why does it mean holding onto all your faculties—and making them even sharper—as you age?

Build an Ageless Mind

Do you know what your body's number-one energy hog is? It's not your muscles, your hard-pumping heart, or even your ever-rumbling belly. It's your brain. After all, if there isn't enough coffee in the control tower, the whole airport shuts down. Likewise, if your bodily control tower runs into a chronic energy shortage, it just might forget to send out the signal to do important stuff like go to work, pay the mortgage, or breathe. So when your body experiences a void between meals, it burns the fat stores in your front porch to keep the lights on upstairs. But on the 8-Hour Diet, it's not just your body that's changing.

Taking time between meals puts your brain to the test, as well. Go back to Dr. Mattson's analogy of intermittent fasting as exercise for the brain. When you exercise, your muscles build new cells to better accommodate the challenges they're being asked to meet. Your brain does the same thing. It meets the challenge posed by energy restriction by increasing the number of cells and synapses available for processing information. Think again of the brain as the control tower of your own personal airport. When there's the threat of a strike by air-traffic controllers, you hire more of them to fill the need to land all those planes safely. The 8-Hour Diet makes sure there are plenty of fresh recruits to handle the mental workload.

The result of all that brain exercise? The snappiest synapses this side of Stephen Hawking. If there was a Tour de Smarts, you'd be tested for steroids. Just look at how you'll benefit:

- **THE 8-HOUR DIET** *may help you create more brain cells and link them together more closely.* You know how, when you're scanning those clues in the crossword puzzle, and suddenly "Terrible, isn't he?" leads you to the only possible answer: "Ivan"? That mental click is what happens when a neuron—a brain cell—sends a spark across a synapse—the connecting point—to another neuron and comes up with a Eureka! moment. The better your neurons and brain cells function, and the more of them there are, the smarter you'll be. And the benefits can extend far beyond 34 Down. Here's what happens, according to Dr. Mattson. When you cut back on food supply on a regular schedule, your brain starts producing more of a miracle protein called *brain-derived neurotrophic factor*—BNDF; having higher levels of this protein helps promote the growth and survival of brain cells. And recently it's been discovered that BNDF can even spur stem cells in your brain tissue to sprout brand-spanking-new cells, which are in turn ready to lock in memories and learn new stuff. The reasoning behind it: A keen mind is more likely to find its way to the next meal. So the downside of not eating leads directly to the upside of clearer thinking. BNDF is also active in strengthening your synapses, so none of your bright ideas get lost in yawning gaps between brain cells (that's the airhead problem, in a nutshell). And it also minimizes brain damage over time, because it produces its own form of antioxidants, which protect your gray matter from the destructive effects of burning energy.

- **THE 8-HOUR DIET** *can protect you from the Big Three of Brain Destroyers.* In their understated way, the Johns Hopkins researchers write that, because of the protective processes kicked off by intermittent fasting, "these dietary regimes could have a significant benefit for debilitating and prevalent neurodegenerative disorders such as Alzheimer's, Huntington's, and Parkinson's diseases." Limiting your time period for caloric intake just seems to make the mind stay sharper as it grows older. "The effect was first shown in rats 30 years ago," says Dr. Mattson. "They looked at calorie-restricted animals' cognitive function, in their ability to solve mazes. Particularly as they got older, the calorie-restricted animals did much better." In fact, there are a number of ways this program protects the brain as it ages . . .

- **THE 8-HOUR DIET** *can fight the inflammation at the heart of Alzheimer's.* Over and above the brain-protective effects I mentioned above, intermittent fasting battles inflammation all over your body. And when it extends that benefit to your brain, it just might help you sidestep Alzheimer's; inflammation is thought to be among the culprits behind it.

- **THE 8-HOUR DIET** *can lessen the effects of stress.* Consider a study published in the *American Journal of Clinical Nutrition* in 2007 that noted that people who kept their food intake to an 8-hour period experienced a "significant decrease in concentrations of cortisol." Cortisol is the hormone your body manufactures when it's under stress, and it tells your body to store fat. Stop stress, and you put a damper on the body's fat-storage mechanism—not to mention the mechanism that causes you to yell at the TV. Another reason to control stress: It's been shown to damage, even destroy, brain cells. But the 8-Hour Diet gives your brain a protective advantage. In his own lab work, Dr. Mattson says, he found that among the benefits of this type of eating plan is "increased production of nerve cell growth factors. It not only encouraged the growth of neurons but also reduced the reaction of neurons to stress."

- **THE 8-HOUR DIET** *can help you avoid having a stroke or recover faster if you do have one.* Losing my own father to stroke at a relatively young age has kept me ever vigilant for new research that can help prevent others from suffering the same fate. Fortunately, the same artery-clearing benefit from intermittent fasting that lowers risk of heart disease can also reduce your risk of stroke. Two albatrosses, one stone. And as anyone with a family history of stroke knows, what doesn't kill us doesn't necessarily make us stronger: A stroke can leave you both physically and mentally disabled. But when scientists intentionally injured the brains of laboratory mice, they found that those on intermittent fasts recovered faster.

- **THE 8-HOUR DIET** *can help you understand the science behind the 8-Hour Diet.* I love the concept of "neuroplasticity," which calls to mind a little kid snapping together plastic Lego blocks to build his dream castle. In fact, it's not that far from the truth, because this concept refers to the brain's miraculous ability to grow, develop, and change all through our lifetime. Neuroplasticity's golden age is childhood, when little ones are using the adaptive and developmental powers of their brain cells to learn how to walk, speak, operate the iPad, and manipulate mom and dad into buying them a smartphone. But neuroplasticity is also a godsend for adults, playing a key role in late-life learning. Intermittent fasting is a great way to have more of it. Why? Because, for mammals like us, hunting for food was a problem that called for creative solutions. ("Hey, maybe there's something gooey and delicious inside that shell. I think I'll invent the oyster knife to pry it open and create cocktail sauce to make it taste better!") So when hunger strikes, your brain's answer is to increase neuroplasticity, both to come up with new ideas for finding food (fried butter on a stick!) and to remember where you found it last year (the Minnesota State Fair!). You'll be able to do more of both on this diet—two things no diet has ever offered before.

• **THE 8-HOUR DIET** *can help you remember all of the benefits of the 8-Hour Diet.* A couple of years ago, a reporter from the *Daily Mail*, in the UK, called up Dr. Mattson to ask him if intermittent fasting could help slow learners speed up. I'll take his response as a resounding yes: "Part of this [learning] effect is due to what cutting calories does to appetite hormones such as ghrelin and leptin," he told the reporter. "When you are not overweight, these hormones encourage growth of new brain cells, especially in the hippocampus. This is the area of the brain that is involved in laying down memories. If you start putting on weight, levels of ghrelin drop and brain cell replacement slows." Then he dropped the hammer: "The effect is particularly damaging in your 40s and 50s, for reasons that aren't clear yet," he says. "Obesity at that age is a marker for cognitive problems later."

You're coming through loud and clear, Dr. Mattson. He'd never say it, but I can: It's quite possible that, as your belly shrinks, your brain grows. And the 8-Hour Diet maximizes that effect.

A buff body and a buff brain? And you can have both while eating whatever you want, as much as you want? No wonder every scientist we spoke to who's investigated this plan has started following it himself or herself. But while you could enjoy all the brain and body benefits of this eating plan even if you took up residence inside a Waffle House, there are ways to turbocharge the effects of the 8-Hour Diet—to add in a set of foods (we call them the 8-Hour Powerfoods) that are so perfectly packed with the right nutrients that they'll help you burn fat even faster and bolster your brainpower even further. We'll explore them in depth in Chapter 5.

At the end of our visit, Dr. Mattson lets fly about a mission he has undertaken with his fast friend Satchidananda Panda, PhD, the Salk Institute scientist who presides over those lucky, skinny, healthy mice who were the first to benefit from an 8-hour diet. According to these bicoastal big brains, it's not enough to write a book about the plan. Now it's time to prescribe intermittent fasting.

"It's getting to the point scientifically that we think it should be incorporated into the medical education curriculum, and that there should be prescriptions that should be given to patients that could be followed up on using social media."

Twitter to make you fitter, in other words.

"One of the big problems with people not being able to stay on a diet is very simple," Dr. Mattson concludes. "It's a psychological thing. Maybe people aren't getting enough encouragement, not getting enough support."

Well, consider that problem over. You can sign up for our feed right now, at Twitter.com/8HourDiet. Why wait for the prescription when you can start tapping into your extended-release life plan and minimized waistline right now?

And by the way, the drive away from Dr. Mattson and the National Institute of Aging was much easier. It always is, when you know your way past the major obstacles and the best way to arrive safely at your destination.

Reset Your Biorhythms to Skinny

Use your natural hormonal clock to maximize the 8-Hour Diet effect!

Would you rather be shaped like an alarm clock or an hourglass?

Up until the beginning of the 20th century, human life operated according to a natural system of biorhythms. We slept when it got dark, and we awoke when it got light. And as a result, our bodies worked within the parameters of our hormonal cycles. Everything proceeded along with our natural circadian rhythms.

And then some wiseguy named Edison came along and screwed it all up.

Nowadays, we can stay up as late as we want, hitting the bar scene, watching *Law & Order* marathons, stalking exes on Facebook, or bathing in the neon glow of our Kindle. Modern life has a lot of advantages. But it has its disadvantages, as well. And one of those disadvantages is that it's screwing up our natural biorhythms, and as a result, it's making us fat. Our reliable body clocks have been turned into time bombs.

According to scientists at the Salk Institute, your eating schedule controls your metabolism. Because we once lived in nighttime darkness, with no automatic refrigerator door light to illuminate our midnight snack, our bodies adapted to a very simple hormonal cycle of work-eat-play-sleep, and our metabolisms burned hot to fuel that schedule. But today, our cycle is more like eat-work-eat-play-eat-eat-sleep-wake up in the middle of the night and eat again.

Research shows that our bodies' inner eat-and-sleep clocks have been thrown completely out of whack, thanks to all-day food cues and too much nighttime artificial light. The result: You're caught in a "fat cycle": a constant flow of hunger hormones that makes you prone to cravings. But when you confine those eating cues to an 8-hour period, you can finally say good-bye to your belly—and stop feeling hungry all the time.

It's all about managing your day to manipulate your hormonal levels. Intermittent fasting has a profound effect on the hunger (ghrelin) and satiety (leptin) hormones. According to the latest endocrine science, it can calm your food cravings and hunger pangs from within, and set you up for weight-loss success. But you've got to manage your meal plan to make that happen. Follow this hour-by-hour slim-down schedule to control hunger hormones, banish cravings, and get trim and toned—fast!

6 TO 8 AM
GET MOVING

Within a half hour of rising, work some movement into your day. (Chapter 10 will give you plenty of options.) Research has found that early morning exercise may help you burn fat more efficiently, and as you know, that effect is compounded by the mechanisms that kick in with intermittent fasting. If you can get outside, even better. Early morning sunlight helps your body naturally reset itself to a healthier sleep/wake cycle (regular indoor lights don't have the same effect). There's no need to do rigorous exercise; a simple walk to the corner store and back will do. You're only trying to elevate your metabolism and burn a few additional calories to work through your glycogen stores and start burning body fat.

6:55 TO 8:55 AM
DRINK UP

Drink at least two 8-ounce glasses of water after rising. Research shows that people who drank this amount lost 5 pounds more than nonguzzlers.

7 TO 9 AM
POWER THROUGH

A lot of 8-Hour Dieters will elect to make lunch their break-fast meal. But if you're in the habit of eating first thing, that could be a challenge—at least initially. But habits—especially unhealthy ones—are meant to be broken. Experience with our test panel tells us that your first day skipping breakfast may be difficult; within 2 weeks, it becomes a lot easier. By the end of the first month, most testers said that skipping breakfast became a painless routine. You may even feel more energized than you did taking on a load of pancakes or soggy muffins and fueling the sugar high/crash cycle. Chapter 9 has a hundred suggestions that will see you through to success in recalibrating your morning cycles.

Reset Your Biorhythms to Skinny

Continued

10 TO 11 AM
HELP YOURSELF TO A HOT BEVERAGE

The hunger and thirst centers of the brain are both located in the hypothalamus, which causes more than a little confusion. If you mistake thirst for hunger, you might wander into the path of the nearest cheeseburger, and it won't be pretty. So drink on a schedule. If you plan for a hot tea or coffee break midmorning, you'll keep your mouth busy, plus warm liquids will make you feel full, longer.

12 TO 1 PM
HOORAY! HAVE YOUR MIDDAY MEAL!

But do it the smart way. Galanin, another hunger hormone that makes you crave fat, rises around lunchtime. However, there's a bit of a vicious (and viscous) cycle here: Eating dietary fat causes you to produce more galanin, which then tells you to eat more fat. Instead, fill up with complex carbs and protein, such as chicken-vegetable soup or black bean chili. In Chapter 5, I'll introduce you to the 8-Hour Powerfoods and show you how having just one serving of each of the 8 Powerfoods (and it's easy—a turkey, tomato, and Swiss on whole wheat gets you halfway there) will ensure a day of perfect nutrition. Make a smart choice at lunch and you'll be on your way to the triumphant cry of "I ate my eight!" (Just close the door to your office before you shout that, OK?) And don't forget: The break-fast meal is set up by the food-free period before it. You'll savor what you eat, and your body will make the most of it as well.

2 TO 3 PM
TAKE A NAP

Instead of hitting the vending machines, find a quiet place to grab a few Zzzs. (Hint: Your parked car is the perfect impromptu sleep pod!) Just set an alarm—15 to 20 minutes will energize your body without affecting your ability to sleep at night. In fact, studies show that midafternoon nappers return to their tasks energized and alert and outperform their groggy peers. Sweet dreams, sweet accomplishments!

3:30 PM
GET BUZZED
Need a boost? This is your last chance to have a cup of joe. Drinking coffee after 4 PM disturbs circadian rhythms and can keep you from falling asleep at night.

4 TO 8 PM
TRIM AND TONE
Now's the ideal time to do your strength training, plus any additional cardio. This is when your body temperature is highest, so you're primed for peak performance. In one study, subjects who worked out in the late afternoon or early evening built 22 percent more muscle than morning exercisers.

5 TO 7 PM
TIME TO DINE
To ensure you don't wake up hungry in the middle of the night, add a serving of healthy fats, such as flaxseed or fish oil, to your meal. If you're a wine drinker, pour a glass now. Drinking later can delay dream (REM) sleep, waking you frequently during the night.

8 TO 9 PM
HAVE A PRESLEEP SNACK, BEFORE YOUR 16-HOUR FAST
Enjoy a carb-based bedtime snack, such as a serving of low-fat frozen yogurt. Nighttime carbs create tryptophan, which helps your brain produce serotonin. This feel-good chemical triggers your body to make melatonin, the sleep hormone.

9 TO 10:30 PM
POWER DOWN
Step away from digital devices, including the TV. They emit a blue spectrum of light that's even more disruptive to sleep than regular bulbs. Do something calming—read, take a bath—in dim light so you're ready to nod off when you hit the sheets.

GO TO SLEEP
9:30 TO 11 PM
Crawl under the covers at the same time each night and wake up at the same time each morning, even on weekends. Having a regular sleep-and-wake schedule helps you fall asleep faster over time, and it helps reset your metabolism to skinny, the 8-Hour Diet way.

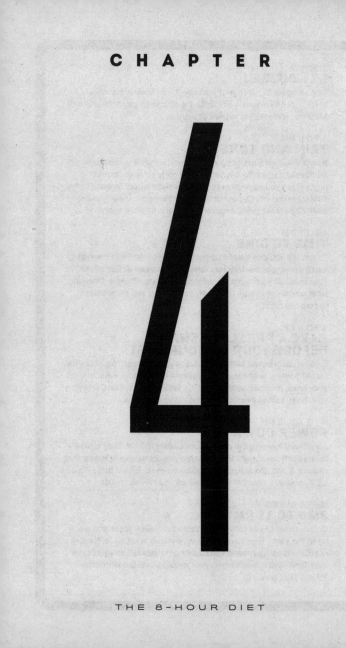

Fast Questions, Fast Answers

Discover just how simple this plan can be!

I've been working as a health journalist for more than half my life. You name an issue—absorption rates of minerals, causes of metabolic syndrome, funding for prostate cancer research, omega-3 versus omega-6 ratios—and if it has something to do with health or wellness, I'll usually have the background on it. I'm not the world's top expert on everything, but chances are, I know the world's top expert.

I'm able to stay on top of stuff because new scientific thinking doesn't usually come out of nowhere. Sure, sometimes during the course of human events an apple falls on a guy's head and he's like, *Whoa, gravity!* But most of the *Holy cow, the Earth is round!* stuff has already been figured out. Nowadays, most breakthroughs in the realm of health and fitness aren't really breakthroughs at all. They're just evolutions of conventional wisdom.

That's why the 8-Hour Diet is so exciting to me. It really does turn conventional wisdom on its head, with an undeniable body of evidence that will change the way we look at nutrition and weight loss, heart disease, diabetes, cancer, and brain diseases.

But this is such a paradigm shift that a lot of folks have a lot of questions—from regular people we talk to about it to the experts at *Men's Health, Women's Health,* and *Prevention* magazines who work with me on a daily basis. Indeed, when we recruited 2,000 people to road-test the 8-Hour Diet, we were bombarded with more questions than a guest star on *Law & Order.* People want to know: Why is this so different from old-fashioned diet plans? And more important, how can it work so well?

In this chapter, I've rounded up some of the most common questions—questions you yourself may share—and explain in detail just what happens when you follow the 8-Hour Diet.

Do I have to eat in the same 8-hour time span every day?

Not at all. The 8-Hour Diet can be easily adapted to any sort of hectic, changing lifestyle. The key to success is simply to alternate 8 hours of feasting with 16 hours of fasting. As long as you stick to that pattern, you'll realize all the benefits.

So, for example, a 9-to-5 type can break her fast at 11 am and be home in time to eat dinner at 7. Presto, that's 8 hours, and she can follow that pattern from week to week. But if a work event, dinner date, or party arises, she can just shift that first meal later in the day, so the 8 hours are 1 pm to 9 pm. And of course, many of us are shift workers who may need to eat our first meal at noon on one day and at 5 pm on another. Fortunately, the plan still works, as long as you observe the 8-hour feasting pattern.

I only want to follow the plan 3 days a week. Should I do my 3 days all in a row, or is it better to alternate them?

Whatever is most convenient for you. For example, some people say they find it easier to wake up late on Saturday and Sunday, enjoy a leisurely morning, and then eat a delicious brunch around noon. (These folks obviously do not have kids.) If that fits your lifestyle, then just slip in one more day during the workweek and you're all set. But if your weekends are hectic, you might want to forget about trying to follow the diet and instead do it Monday, Tuesday, Wednesday. Or Monday, Wednesday, Friday. Or Tuesday, Wednesday, Thursday. Or whatever. As long as you hit your times, you'll change your body—and your life.

Can I eat as often as I want during my 8 hours?

Yes! You're free to eat what you like, when you like. If you want two big meals at lunch and dinner and that's it, fine. If you want to graze through the whole 8 hours, that's okay, too. It really depends on your lifestyle and your favorite foods.

Am I allowed to have coffee or tea during the fasting period? And can I put milk and sugar in it, or is that cheating?

Coffee and tea are absolutely encouraged because caffeine is an appetite suppressant. But it's also a mild diuretic, so make sure you're taking extra fluids to compensate. As for the milk and sugar: Yes, that's cheating, but your secret is safe with us. It's a minor intake of calories, but if it makes your favorite beverage go down easier, go for it. Just try to keep the additions as light as possible.

Can I have milk, juice, soda, sweetened coffee drinks, or bottled iced teas during the fasting period?

Hell no.

There's really only one way to screw up this diet, and it's by drinking lots of extra calories during your fasting times. And it's an easy mistake to make. The average American drinks a whopping 450 calories a day, and many of them come from surprising sources.

For example, let's say you want to stay hydrated during your fast, so you reach for a bottle of flavored water—in this case, Snapple Tropical Mango Antioxidant Water. What could be bad about that? It's got antioxidants, for goodness sake! But in fact you're drinking 150 calories of pure sugar along with your H_2O. Drinking just one of these concoctions a day in place of plain water will add 15 pounds to your body over the course of a year. And worse, you've broken your fast with these junk calories, so bye-bye health and weight-loss benefits! For the maximum benefit, stick with calorie-free drinks.

I'm a competitive runner. Is this diet suitable for athletes or for other people who work out regularly?
It's not only suitable, it's encouraged. The fat-burning effects of fasting will be multiplied by strong workouts. Look at it this way: The NBA Hall-of-Famer Hakeem Olajuwon regularly fasted during the basketball season. He was once named "player of the month" during February, when he fasted for Ramadan. If he could play that well at an elite level while fasting, you can, too.

What if I need a snack?
Hunger and thirst are both registered in the hypothalamus, so when you're tempted to eat, have a drink instead. Hot tea. Iced tea. Sparkling water with lime. Pick your favorite no-cal beverage and tank up. Your belly will be full, and the hunger will pass.

Am I really allowed to eat as much as I want during my 8 hours? I have a pretty large appetite.
Yes and no. Live your life as you see fit. But if you expect to have results on this diet plan, don't go crazy on us—slow down, and eat until you're sated, not stuffed. Unless you substantially increase the amount of food you're eating each day—hard to do that as long as you're eating within the prescribed time period—you're going to see dramatic results. But why not use this plan as a reason to reconsider consumption? Stay within the boundaries of the 8-Hour Powerfoods and the 8 hours. It could be the start of a whole new you.

Everything I've read about weight loss says I shouldn't skip breakfast—how can fasting in the morning be healthy?

There are plenty of ways to lose weight, and eating a solid, high-protein breakfast is one of them. But it isn't the only way. We know from all of the studies we've gathered that the 8-Hour Diet will help you lose weight, regardless of when your 8 hours begins and ends.

Skipping breakfast is how most of the experts we've spoken to prefer to manage their own weight, but you're free to schedule your feeding and fasting times however you like. So if it's easier for you, logistically, to break your fast at 8 am and eat until 4 pm, go for it. And there is an advantage there, because the end of your fast will come when you're asleep. Plus, the classic breakfast foods—eggs, bacon, yogurt, whole-wheat toast, oatmeal—give you plenty of nutritional support. But fasting in the morning has its advantages, as well. Dinner is often the most sociable meal of the day, and you'll probably want to join your loved ones at the table. Pick the daily schedule that works best for you, and enjoy your success!

Can I have a cheat day?

You can have four cheat days a week if you want. Following the 8-Hour Diet 7 days a week is hard to do, so I tell most folks to try it 3 to 5 days a week for starters. Four cheat days will still work for you, promise!

But "cheat days" does not mean "strap yourself to the all-you-can-eat-buffet-until-you-pass-out days." Try to make sure you "eat your 8" even on days when you're not following the diet to ensure that you're getting all the nutrition you need, and be smart about your food choices.

I keep long hours, and I like to incorporate a protein shake or small snack before my early morning workout. Can I still have my shake or does that count as breaking the fast?

Yes, you'd be breaking the fast, but then this plan is yours to design and retrofit in a way that works for your life. So if there's no way to accommodate that protein shake along with your workout into your 8-hour eating period, go ahead and break the rules. But bear this in mind, as well: All the scientific evidence points to a strict fast as the best way to achieve maximum results. So the first, best option is to keep the fast; the second best option is to live your life as you need to and be as careful with your 8/16 pattern as possible.

I've been told that you have to eat frequently to retain muscle mass. If I fast, won't I lose muscle?

No, you won't. Quite the contrary. One of the most surprising aspects of intermittent fasting is that it forces your body to burn fat preferentially instead of muscle.

This is one factor that dramatically sets the 8-Hour Diet apart from other diet plans. Typically, reducing caloric intake—your standard "crash" diet—causes the body to burn muscle for energy. In the long run, that causes your metabolism to slow down, meaning that once you go off your crash diet, you wind up fatter than before you started it. This is why so many celebrities are walking examples of so-called "yo-yo dieting"—they dramatically lose weight for a role or photo shoot, but they come back bigger than ever, and not in a good way.

Why is the 8-Hour Diet different? Among the first pieces of anecdotal evidence that researchers in this field began noticing was how popular fasting had become in the bodybuilding community: It worked to help the overly buff achieve that cut, muscular look that won competitions—and didn't erode muscle size or quality. In fact, muscle strength and athletic performance seemed to improve. While the exact mechanism is still being studied, we do know that intermittent fasting increases natural levels of human growth hormone, or HGH—the stuff that aging athletes inject illegally to help them stay young and strong.

What it means to you: Limiting your food consumption to 8 hours a day triggers your body to burn fat for energy; standard dieting leads you to burn muscle. Take your pick.

Doesn't fasting cause your metabolism to slow down?

No. It will actually accelerate it. If it didn't, our species (and other carnivores like us) would never have survived into the modern era.

Think of it: Your ancient ancestor is out cruising the plains of Africa during a time of food shortages. She's hungry and needs a meal. If her metabolism slowed down, she wouldn't be able to chase the prey she spots down by the water hole. But she is up for that chase, because her body, metabolically primed for the hunt, is burning stored fat in the absence of food, just like yours is on the 8-Hour Diet. Her pattern of feasting and fasting, just like yours, also maintains muscle mass—it aids in the hunt but also boosts metabolism for the big charge. Sure, if you try to live on rice cakes, grapefruit, and Diet Coke for days on end, your metabolism will slow down—the fatal flaw of traditional diets. But that won't happen on this plan. You should eat good food, and plenty of it—but just within the allotted 8 hours.

Don't our bodies store fat in response to periods of hunger?

No, but they do store fat in response to standard dieting. Here's why. When you go on a standard diet, you may lose weight initially. But when your body senses that there's a real dearth of food available—when you go day after day taking in fewer calories than your body needs—all that deprivation sets off a kind of hormonal panic in your body. Your body starts to reduce its production of leptin, the hormone that suppresses appetite, and boost levels of ghrelin, the hormone that encourages hunger. You become famished because your body wants you to go into calorie-storage mode.

So now you've got overwhelming signals of hunger, thanks to your hormonal system. Plus, when you do give in and hit the buffet, your body is primed to store those calories as fat, because it's been told by your "diet" that food is scarce, and it might be a long time before you eat again, so you'd better pack on some easy-to-store, slow-to-burn fat. And you'd better hold on to that fat no matter what!

Intermittent fasting, however, isn't based on deprivation. It's a pattern of eating, not purgatory, and it reinforces to your body that it will get plenty of healthy calories every day so there's no reason to store fat—in fact, it can start burning fat for energy. Studies show that it also causes a surge in hunger-limiting leptin. So if you really want to ditch the weight, ditch the diet and change your eating schedule instead.

What's the difference between "intermittent fasting" and "caloric restriction" or "disordered eating"? Am I setting myself up for an eating disorder?

Absolutely not. First, the definitions, which will help you understand why the 8-Hour Diet is just about the opposite of an eating disorder.

Intermittent fasting is a regularly scheduled, planned abstinence from food. There are lots of ways to do it: Some people do it one day a week or on special occasions, not eating from sundown one day until sundown the following day— the common method in religious observance. Others follow a method called alternate-day fasting, which is just what it sounds like. And then there's the 8-Hour Diet, in which you eat for a set time period—it's the easy way to accomplish the same goals.

Caloric restriction means routinely consuming a fraction of the normal food and energy intake to maintain your health; if the standard diet for a woman is 1,800 calories, restrictors would take in 1,100 or so. It's also known as the "perpetual suffering" diet and is very hard to stick to. Disordered eating refers to an out-of-control pattern of bingeing and starving, often under psychological duress; bulimia and anorexia nervosa are examples. Eating disorders are emotionally and psychologically driven and wouldn't be "caused" by intermittent fasting, which is, by its nature, a controlled pattern of eating. Disordered eaters have no control over their eating patterns; that's why they need to seek psychological counseling to regain control.

I get woozy when my blood sugar gets low, and I'm often told it's because I didn't eat. Will I pass out from fasting?

Everyone should have a primary-care physician who knows their general eating and exercise patterns. Before you undertake any major change, it makes sense to talk to your doctor first. That's especially true if you have a blood-sugar disorder—diabetes or pre-diabetes, for instance—in which case you can run into trouble if you are restricting food intake or altering your eating patterns.

For the rest of us, however, there is always sufficient glycogen stored in the liver to meet immediate energy needs; if you do burn through that, the body switches to burning fat.

I've been sticking to the fast, but sometimes I get hungry before it's time to eat. Any tips for how I can curb the cravings during my fasting window?

The key to sticking with the fast when you're hungry: distraction. Don't sit still, obsessing about food. Get on your feet. Take a walk. Visit a coworker for a chat about some big project you're working on. Watch a funny video on YouTube. Then watch another. Go for a workout. Run an errand. Most hunger pangs last 10 minutes at most, so occupy your body and mind for that length of time, and often the hunger will simply pass. (Check out Chapter 9 for a hundred such strategies for curbing cravings.) Also keep in mind: You'll get better at this as the weeks go by, so stick with it now, and you'll master it soon enough!

Can I still take my usual vitamins and supplements while I'm fasting?

Go for it.

What if I need to skip a week?

The 8-Hour Diet is all about the real world. So during your week off, see if you can keep to it on a modified basis, say 10 hours of eating, 14 of fasting. Do your best while you're off the wagon, then clamber back on as soon as possible. In fact, this diet is very flexible; if you stick with it most of the time, you'll receive benefits most of the time as well. The closer you are to 8/16, the better it'll work. But it's not a failure if you aren't quite up to that mark.

I'm a vegetarian/vegan. How can I make the 8-Hour Diet work for me?

First of all, congratulations. You're starting from a better place than the rest of us omnivores. Simply adapt the eight Powerfoods as needed. Obviously, you won't be eating meat, so use your best protein swaps to meet that category. Ditto the bean-curd variations (soy milk) for dairy, if you're not doing the cow thing. Otherwise, you're good to go green and still get lean.

TURN ANY DIET INTO AN 8-HOUR DIET

**How to take your favorite weight-loss plans
and make them even better**

T he worst thing about the diet-book industry: If you go with the most popular eating plan of the moment, you'll be changing your diet as often as most teenagers change their socks. In with the Lemonade Diet, out with the Brown Fat Revolution. But wait, here comes the Cookie Diet. If only there were a Glass of Milk Diet to go along with it!

In a funny way, that's exactly the point I want to make here: Synergy can work. In fact, the best, most popular weight-loss plans out there—the Atkins Diet, the Paleo Diet, the South Beach Diet, Wheat Belly, and my own Abs Diet and Eat This, Not That! franchises—have gained fans for really good reasons: They make sense, they work, and people can stick with them. But new research emerges, eating habits change, and readers often find they have to abandon what works for them in order to follow the new science.

Until now, that is.

The 8-Hour Diet can actually make any of these top-flight plans even better. How? Look at it this way: Each of the plans mentioned above proposes a sensible eating program based on solid science. But none of them takes advantage of the profound biological mechanisms that kick in with intermittent fasting. So, what if you inserted a best-selling diet into an 8-hour eating plan? You'll get the best of both worlds—and they're both populated by skinny, healthy people!

Here's how you can work it.

THE 8-HOUR ATKINS

THE ATKINS DIET, IN A NUTSHELL: Shun carbs, vegetables, and fruits and welcome back all the animal fats and proteins you'd been taught to avoid.

THE DOWNSIDES: Yes, you can even get sick of bacon, plus you miss out on the valuable mitochondria-repairing antioxidants you get from fruit, vegetables, and whole grains. (Sadly, you won't be able to "eat your 8" if you're following Atkins.)

THE 8-HOUR ANGLE: While I don't recommend it fully, if you do follow Atkins, you'll find that the 8-Hour Diet will turbocharge its effects. And there's a double benefit here: 1) The protein and fats prescribed by Dr. Atkins (may he rest in hog heaven) have a built-in satiety effect, so they'll sustain you during your fasting period; and 2) some researchers worry about increased heart-disease and stroke risk on an all-meat diet. Well, voilà, the cardio- and brain-protective benefits of the 8-Hour Diet just might save you from an Atkins attack. So if you eat every part of the pig but the oink, your 8-hour eating schedule just might protect you in the long run.

THE 8-HOUR CAVEMAN

THE PALEO DIET, IN A NUTSHELL: Never eat anything our caveman forebears wouldn't have eaten back in Paleolithic times. Out with the processed foods, grains, legumes, and carbs, in with the brontosaurus burgers (sans roll), tree nuts, fruits, whole vegetables, line-caught fish, and lean meats.

THE DOWNSIDES: All that focus on excluding what our caveman forebears didn't eat leaves out a whole bunch of delicious and beneficial foods they might have benefited from, including low-fat dairy, beans, and whole grains. Cavemen didn't have painless dentistry either, so it's not like progress is always a bad thing.

THE 8-HOUR ANGLE: Again, let's scrunch down all that good, prehistoric eating into 8 hours and leave all the sugar and refined carbs to soon-to-be extinct, unenlightened modern men and women. (Grunt if you like that.) But you can also build in an "I ate my 8!" angle here, so you have the benefit of whole grains and dairy while not straying too far off the Paleo plan. The best part: Adding those two categories neatly rounds out the caveman menu, which means you'll be able to stay on the diet while other knuckle-draggers fall by the wayside. And the longer you stick with any diet, the more likely you are to lock in its benefits.

8 HOURS ON SOUTH BEACH

THE SOUTH BEACH DIET, IN A NUTSHELL: *The South Beach Diet's* Dr. Agatston is a world-renowned cardiologist, so his goal has been not just weight loss, but heart health as well. He seized on some aspects of his colleague Dr. Atkin's plan and civilized it considerably. It was no longer just bacon for bacon's sake, but rather, that South Beach cuts carbs radically and replaces them with a wholesome foods plan that includes healthy grains, fruits, and vegetables and broadens the protein appeal to fatty fishes and dairy. This was Atkins for Miami models, and the masses descended upon it.

THE LIMITATIONS: There isn't much to disagree with, although an exercise program should be a part of any South Beach weight-loss plan.

THE 8-HOUR ANGLE: Dr. Agatston's delicious and healthful food recommendations look even better on an 8-hour eating schedule, because now you have both sides of the boat rowing in the same direction: Four food oars pulling toward great nutrition for health and weight-loss benefits, four fasting oars pulling for the brain, heart, and cancer-fighting benefits. And it adds up to eight! What's more, you'll have a megadose of insulin management: Both the South Beach Diet and the 8-Hour eating plan can profoundly affect the way your body processes blood sugar, so this is an antidiabetes double play, as well.

THE 8-HOUR WHEAT BELLY BUSTER

WHEAT BELLY, IN A NUTSHELL: If I were a carb, I'd be getting nervous. For as hard as Drs. Atkins and Agatston were on carbs, Dr. William Davis is all that and no bag of chips. He banished carbs from Planet You and has been shrinking equators across the land ever since. *Wheat Belly* recommends plenty of nuts and vegetables, but also plenty of fat, to keep the stomach growling to a minimum.

THE LIMITATIONS: As with Atkins, even healthy grains like oatmeal are banished from the island, as well as other healthy foods (like fruit, legumes and beans, and gluten-free grains).

THE 8-HOUR ANGLE: Cutting out wheat has a lot of benefits, and once you read what Dr. Davis has to say about the genetic game of Twister that scientists have played with the grain's DNA, you'll happily pass on the bread basket. *Wheat Belly* focuses on reducing insulin resistance and diabetes risk, benefits that you'll optimize if you follow the plan in combination with the 8-Hour Diet. Bonus for all of you who are concerned about celiac disease: Intermittent fasting has been shown to be a potent way to battle autoimmune disorders, and celiac has many autoimmune characteristics.

THE 8-HOUR NEW ABS DIET

THE NEW ABS DIET, IN A NUTSHELL: I created this program, too, so forgive me if I indulge it like a parent. It's hard to see its flaws when it's of your own flesh—and less of it, at that. Build your diet around the ABS DIET POWER foods (Almonds, Beans, Spinach, Dairy, Instant oatmeal, Eggs, Turkey, Peanut butter, Olive oil, Whole grains, Extra-protein powder, Raspberries—and like foods), supplement your meals with high-protein smoothies, and build your workouts around muscle-building fat burners. You hit your middle from both sides and slim your way to a six-pack.

THE LIMITATIONS: The nutrition and exercise principles in the *New Abs Diet* are as sound as the day I wrote them, but the new research about the importance of when you eat—as opposed to just what you eat—was only beginning to percolate to the surface.

8-HOUR ABS: Doesn't that sound awesome? And it's not a dream, either. In fact, the fat-burning properties of the feast and fast cycle, combined with the high-protein smoothie recipes and workouts, might generate more six-packs than the Budweiser plant in St. Louis. Pick one up!

EAT THIS, NOT THAT FOR 8 HOURS

EAT THIS, NOT THAT! IN A NUTSHELL: Not a diet plan at all, *Eat This, Not That!* has helped people lose 10, 20, 30—sometimes up to 100 pounds—just by eating the same foods, but healthier, lower-calorie versions of them. The idea is that you can keep going to Wendy's for lunch, keep grabbing dinner at Red Robin, and keep enjoying takeout from Domino's or from the convenience section of your supermarket, but by knowing which products to buy, you can strip away pounds automatically.

THE LIMITATIONS: While stripping away fat and calories by eating healthier restaurant fare is great, what's even better is cooking at home with fresh, nutrition-packed ingredients. (Fortunately, there are three *Cook This, Not That!* books to choose from!)

THE 8-HOUR ANGLE: Actually, *Eat This, Not That!* is the perfect accompaniment to the 8-Hour Diet. If you shorten the time frame in which you eat, convenience becomes a top priority.

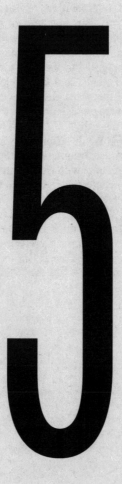

5

The 8 Foods You Should Eat Every Day

Perfect nutrition made easy

A diet that lets me eat all my favorite foods? What's the catch? Well, I want you to keep eating your favorite foods—but I *also* want you to eat these eight superfoods, foods so potent in their nutritional punch that they'll ensure your body is perfectly fueled.

The 8-Hour Diet is the only scientifically proven weight-loss plan that allows you to eat as much as you want of whatever you want. It's one of the most exciting nutritional development since the Aztecs figured out how to make the first chocolate out of cacao beans.

In fact, the only challenge to the 8-Hour Diet is finding time to eat lots of delicious food. (Heck, you should proba-bly put your favorite barbecue joint on speed dial—just so you can satisfy your most gluttonous cravings at the touch of a button!)

But while eating as much as you want of whatever you want is a pretty exciting promise, it doesn't mean you can start living exclusively on Cherry Coke and Doritos. Your body still has some basic nutritional requirements that can't be fully satisfied by the dollar menu at Wendy's. You need good-for-you fats for looking and feeling healthy; you need fiber to keep you full and satisfied; you need vitamins to ward off disease and minerals to pump your blood and move your muscles. And you need variety to make your taste buds happy!

How can you ensure that you're getting all the nutrients your body craves—even while indulging your desire for take-out, fast food, and dessert? To this end, I've identified the 8-Hour Powerfoods—eight food categories, each of which comes with its own treasure trove of nutrients. Simply by eating one serving from each of these categories every day—instead of or *in addition to* anything else you'd like to eat!—you'll ensure perfect nutrition and maximum health. In other words, go nuts at 5 Guys Burgers and Fries tomorrow afternoon, but make sure your next meal or snack contains these nutritional all-stars.

The 8-Hour Powerfoods are, quite simply, the best foods I know. Allow me to introduce you to them. You'll see that they fall into two main categories—the Fat Busters and the Health Boosters. Each category has four food groups under it, and each of those groups contains a groaning banquet table of options, bursting with amazing flavors, textures, aromas, colors, and nutrients. At the end of each day, if you can say "I ate my 8!" then you'll have no question about whether you're fueling your body with the absolute best mix of foods on the planet—no matter what else you ate that day.

The Path to Perfect Nutrition

I've divided the 8-Hour Powerfoods into two categories. One set is made up of rich, delicious foods high in protein, fiber, and healthy fats (the Fat Busters); they'll help your body build and maintain lean muscle, burn off flab, and fend off hunger. Those are complemented by foods high in vitamins and minerals (the Health Boosters) that can help you fight the most common causes of disease and death and sharpen your mind at the same time they help you preserve cherished memories.

(To make it even easier to say "I ate my 8," chef and James Beard Award–nominated food journalist Matt Goulding, my coauthor on the Cook This, Not That! series, has created a bounty of simple and delicious recipes that incorporate the 8-Hour Powerfoods; they're collected in Chapter 8. And you don't need to be Anthony Bourdain or Gordon Ramsay to make these recipes sing—they're as easy as lighting a match, and many can be pulled together in just 8 minutes!)

In fact, you don't have to cook—or even know where your kitchen is—to make every day an 8-Hour Powerfood day. You can grab most of these foods and eat on the run, order them over the counter at your local deli, or even snack on them while you're at the bar watching the game.

To hit the road to maximum health and weight loss as quickly as possible, try to eat at least one or two of the 8-Hour Powerfoods with each snack or meal. By virtue of your 8-Hour eating schedule, your body will already be selectively burning belly fat for calories. These foods will turbocharge that effect as they help you firm up lean muscle mass (which burns more calories) and avoid storing fat in the first place. (Select your new swimsuit now: You'll need it for your coming beach vacation—the one you'll pay for with the money you save on this plan.)

More ways to put the Powerfood jolt in your life:

FIND WAYS TO COMBINE THEM. The recipes in Chapter 8 are a start, but once you become familiar with the groups and find favorites within them, you'll stop making a distinction between "what tastes good" and "what's good for you." Both can be true. Dig in, times eight!

BE THE WARREN BUFFETT OF THE BUFFET. Consider each meal and snack to be an investment in your body. You want to create a balanced portfolio of investments that are going to perform well, and try to cut down on "junk" bonds—investments that aren't a good value. Eating a variety of proteins, complex carbohydrates, and good fats is the best way to satisfy hunger without bingeing, and you'll fulfill all your nutritional requirements at the same time.

EAT ALL THE COLORS OF THE RAINBOW. Nature created fruits and vegetables with their own color-coded branding system. Red fruits and vegetables, for example, are rich in lycopene, which fights heart disease and protects against sun damage. Orange and yellow foods pack lots of vitamin A; greens are high in folate and vitamin K; and blue and purple hues mean the food is high in other nutrients and antioxidants. So if you mix colors, you'll max out on health benefits.

Meet the 8-Hour Powerfoods!

The first criterion I applied when picking the Powerfoods was that they be flat-out delicious. (And if they aren't amazing to begin with, the recipes in Chapter 8 will *make* them delicious!) If foods don't taste great, I don't eat them, and I know you won't either. So consider this a smorgasbord of earthly delights to include in your 8-Hour feast.

But there are other benefits aside from the tickle on the tongue, which is why I call them Powerfoods. All of them have that *Fantastic Voyage*–like ability to travel through the byways of your body and fix what's wrong, or even, *Terminator*-like, to stop an impending future disaster in its tracks, today. Keep clear a crucial artery here, hook up a new brain synapse there, ignite a sexual spark down there, all the while priming your metabolism to burn through belly fat the way John Mayer burns through girlfriends. Isn't it great knowing that just by eating these foods, you're setting up your body for a lifetime of health?

I've arranged a panel of handy icons to tell you exactly where and how eating these foods will help you. Keep in mind that the very fact that you're on the 8-Hour Diet touches off profound biological changes in your body, so you'll be experiencing all of the benefits enumerated below, and more. But now, as you eat your way through the excellent eight, you'll be amplifying and multiplying those benefits.

Eat by the icons *and* by the clock, and you'll enjoy the healthiest heights of your lifetime. Take the 8-Hour Powerfoods home for dinner. Tomorrow morning, you'll want to spend the rest of your life with them.

BUILDS MUSCLE. The 8-Hour Diet will send your blood levels of human growth hormone soaring, so you're already primed to build muscle. Plant and animal proteins—plus certain minerals, such as magnesium—are muscle-building essentials, so they'll give your muscle-building hormones plenty of raw material to work with. And the 8-Minute Workouts will be jacking you up, as well. So much the better if you do frequent drinking-glass curls and fork presses with these muscular foods and libations.

HELPS PROMOTE WEIGHT LOSS. The belly-shrinking benefits of eating for 8 hours a day are already significant. Pack those hours with foods high in calcium and fiber (both of which protect against obesity), plus foods that help build fat-busting muscle tissue, and you're on your way to a lean belly.

 STRENGTHENS BONE. Calcium and vitamin D are the most important bone builders, and they protect the body against osteoporosis. But beware: High levels of sodium can leach calcium out of bone tissue. Fortunately, all of the great eight Powerfoods are naturally low in sodium.

 LOWERS BLOOD PRESSURE. A 2001 study published in the *Journal of Manipulative and Physiological Therapy* (hey, it's on *my* coffee table) showed an *average* blood-pressure drop of 37/13 mm Hg in hypertensive patients who fasted regularly. And now you'll be eating food that's low in sodium *and* has beneficial amounts of potassium, magnesium, or calcium. Your jackrabbit pulse just might slow to tortoise speed—and you'll win the longevity race.

 FIGHTS CANCER. The tumor-taming result of intermittent fasting is among its most remarkable effects. Now you'll also be a living test subject for the abundant research showing a lower cancer risk among those people who maintain low-fat, high-fiber diets. (I'd recommend that you donate your body to science, but perhaps it'll be so sexy you'll want to keep using it yourself.) You can also help foil cancer by eating foods that are high in calcium, beta-carotene, or vitamin C. In addition, all cruciferous (cabbage-type) and allium (onion-type) vegetables can help prevent various types of cancer. They're all here, in the eight Powerfoods.

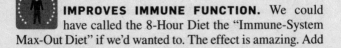 **IMPROVES IMMUNE FUNCTION.** We could have called the 8-Hour Diet the "Immune-System Max-Out Diet" if we'd wanted to. The effect is amazing. Add

a healing dose of vitamins A, E, B_6, and C; folate; and the mineral zinc, and you'll redouble the body's immunity to certain diseases. This icon will lead you to Powerfoods with high levels of one or more of these nutrients.

 FIGHTS HEART DISEASE. When it comes to heart health, the 8-Hour Powerfoods are like nutritional Navy SEALs, targeting and destroying artery-clogging cholesterol by limiting saturated and trans fats and maxing out on foods that are high in monounsaturated or polyunsaturated fats.

The Fat Busters

The first four food groups in our Elite 8 will keep you satisfied long after your jaws stop moving. The reason: They're the dietary equivalent of your handy Uncle Bob, who comes for Thanksgiving dinner and doesn't leave until the filters on your furnace are changed, all the lightbulbs are converted over to compact fluorescents, the spark plugs in the lawn mower have been replaced, and that new closet organizer is installed. Like Uncle Bob, these foods combine staying power, long-lasting energy supplies, and a utility belt that puts the Dark Knight to shame. Invite them over for a long weekend—and the long life that follows.

Turkey, Chicken (and Eggs!), Fish, and Other Lean Meats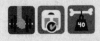

8-HOUR POWERS: Build muscle, burn fat
SECRET WEAPONS: Protein (eggs, especially), iron, zinc, creatine (beef), omega-3 fatty acids (fish), vitamins B_6

(chicken and fish) and B_{12} (eggs, again), phosphorus, potassium, vitamin A

FIGHTS AGAINST: Obesity, hunger pangs, flabby arms
SIDEKICKS: Shellfish, Canadian bacon
IMPOSTERS: Sausage, bacon, cured meats, ham, fatty cuts of steak like T-bone and rib-eye, Egg Beaters, egg-white omelets (why leave out the most nutritionally potent part of the egg?)

A classic muscle-building nutrient, protein is the base of any solid diet plan. That's why this category is such a big and important one. It takes more energy for your body to digest the protein in meat than it does to digest carbohydrates or fat, so the more protein you eat, the more calories you burn. Many studies support the notion that high-protein diets promote weight loss. In one study, researchers in Denmark found that men who substituted protein for 20 percent of their carbs increased their metabolism and increased the number of calories they burned every day by up to 5 percent.

Among your protein sources, turkey is a rare bird. Turkey breast is one of the leanest meats you'll find, and it packs nearly one-third of your daily requirements of niacin and vitamin B_6. Dark meat, if you prefer, has lots of zinc and iron. Two cautions, though: If you're roasting a whole turkey for a family feast, avoid self-basting birds, which have been injected with fat. And avoid eating the skin, which contains most of the fat.

Beef is another classic muscle-building protein. It's the top food source for creatine—the substance your body uses to tone your muscles. Beef does have a downside: It contains saturated fats, but some cuts have more than others. Look for rounds or loins (that's code for extra-lean); sirloins and New York strips are less fatty than prime ribs and T-bones. And choose a smaller portion for your plate, which can help you lose weight without making you feel deprived. For example, by having a 6-ounce steak instead of an 8-ouncer, you'll save 140 calories and still get 46 grams of muscle-building protein. Another tip: Wash down that steak with a glass of milk.

Research shows that calcium may reduce the amount of saturated fat your body absorbs.

Choose cuts from the top of the list that follows. They contain less fat but still pack high amounts of protein.

Fat Content of Meat

4 OZ, RAW, WITHOUT SKIN OR BONE	TOTAL FAT G	SATURATED G
SKINLESS CHICKEN BREAST	1.41	0.37
VEAL STEAK	2.45	0.74
WILD RABBIT	2.63	0.78
LEAN GROUND BEEF	4	1.50
CURED HAM	4.68	1.56
WILD DUCK BREAST	4.82	1.50
CHICKEN DRUMSTICK	5.05	1.34
LEAN PORK TENDERLOIN	5.06	1.79
BEEF SIRLOIN STEAK	5.15	2
BUFFALO	5.44	2.31
TURKEY LEG	7.62	2.34
TURKEY BREAST	7.96	2.17
LEAN BEEF TENDERLOIN	8.02	3
LEAN PORK CHOP	8.19	2.85
PORTERHOUSE STEAK	8.58	3
LEAN GROUND TURKEY	9.37	2.55
VEAL BREAST MEAT	9.73	3.80
RIB-EYE STEAK	18.03	7.30
T-BONE STEAK	19.63	7.69
HAM	21.40	7.42
PORK BELLY	60.11	21.92
CURED PORK	91.29	33.32

The Super Fat

As I hope you learned from the litany of healthy-fat Powerfoods, not all fats are created equal, and olive oil is among the finest of them all. Its superpowers include lowering cholesterol and boosting the immune system, and it amplifies the benefits of the 8-Hour Diet in the fight against obesity, cancer, heart disease, and high blood pressure. (Canola oil, peanut oil, and sesame oil can help, too.) Olive oil and its brethren will help you eat less by controlling your food cravings; they'll also help you burn fat and keep your cholesterol in check.

Do you need any more reason to pass the bottle? Apply by the tablespoon as you sauté and bake (canola oil is especially useful here), displacing the vegetable and hydrogenated oils in your diet, along with scary trans fat and margarine.

To cut down on saturated fats even more, concentrate on getting your protein from fish like tuna, salmon, and sardines, because they contain a healthy dose of omega-3 fatty acids. Omega-3s lower levels of a hormone called leptin in your body. Several recent studies suggest that leptin directly influences your metabolism: The higher your sustained leptin levels, the more readily your body stores calories as fat. Researchers at the University of Wisconsin found that mice with low leptin levels have faster metabolisms and are able to burn fat faster than animals with higher leptin levels. Whether you eat fish or not, consider taking omega-3 supplements.

Which comes first, nutritionally: the chicken or her eggs? I'll put my money on those embryonic chickens, in fact. For a long time, eggs were considered pure evil—more likely to appear in the Most Wanted poster at the post office than in a healthy-eating chapter of a diet book. That's because everybody—including food scientists and health editors—spent several decades in confusion over cholesterol. It was in food, and it was implicated in fatal blood clots in the heart.

Same name, direct link. Right? Wrong. Five decades later it has become clear that food cholesterol and blood cholesterol are different animals and not really related to one another. In fact, we've now learned that most blood cholesterol is made by the body from dietary fat, not dietary cholesterol. And that's why you should take advantage of eggs and their powerful dose of protein. Eggs have the highest "biological value" of protein—a measure of how well it supports your body's protein need—of any food. In other words, egg protein is more effective in building muscle than protein from other sources, even milk and beef. Eggs also contain vitamin B_{12}, which is important for fat breakdown.

Walnuts and Other Nuts

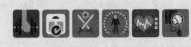

8-HOUR POWERS: Build muscle, fight cravings
SECRET WEAPONS: Protein, monounsaturated fats, vitamin E, fiber, magnesium, folate (peanuts), phosphorus
FIGHTS AGAINST: Obesity, heart disease, muscle loss, wrinkles, cancer
SIDEKICKS: Pumpkin seeds, sunflower seeds, avocados
IMPOSTERS: Salted, candied, or smoked nuts

These days, you hear about good fats and bad fats the way you hear about good cops and bad cops. One's on your side, and one's gonna beat you silly. Oreos fall into the latter category, but nuts are clearly out to help you. They contain the monounsaturated fats that clear your arteries and help you feel full.

All nuts are high in protein and monounsaturated fat. But almonds are the Usain Bolt of nuts: They're undeniably nutty, but they still manage to finish well ahead of the pack. A handful of almonds provides half the amount of vitamin E you need in a day and 8 percent of the calcium. This handful also contains 19 percent of your daily requirement of magnesium—a key component for muscle building. In a

Western Washington University study, people taking extra magnesium were able to lift 20 percent more weight and build more muscle than those who weren't.

A 2009 study in the *American Journal of Clinical Nutrition* showed that eating almonds suppresses hunger, and the more you chew them, the greater your feelings of fullness will be. In the study, people who chewed 25 to 40 times absorbed more healthy monounsaturated fats and had higher levels of appetite-suppressing hormones than those who chewed just 10 times. You can eat as much as two handfuls of almonds a day. A Toronto University study found that men can eat this amount daily without gaining any extra weight. A Purdue University study showed that people who ate nuts high in monounsaturated fat felt full an hour and a half longer than those who ate fat-free food (rice cakes, in this instance). If you eat 2 ounces of almonds (about 24 of them), it should be enough to suppress your appetite—especially if you wash them down with 8 ounces of water. The fluid helps expand the fiber in the nuts to help you feel fuller. Also, try to keep the nuts' nutrient-rich skins on them.

Here are ways to introduce almonds seamlessly into your diet:

- **Add chopped almonds to plain peanut butter.**
- **Toss a handful on cereal, yogurt, or ice cream.**
- **Put slivers in an omelet.**
- **For a quick popcorn alternative: Spray a handful of almonds with nonstick cooking spray for just a fraction of a second, and bake at 400°F for 5 minutes. Take them out of the oven, and sprinkle with either brown sugar and cinnamon or cayenne pepper and thyme.**

But don't stop at almonds. Walnuts, pistachios, Brazil nuts, and pecans also deliver amazing health benefits. No food packs more selenium than Brazil nuts; 1 ounce has almost 10 times the recommended dietary allowance. University of Arizona scientists recently found that selenium may prevent colon cancer in men. Walnuts, on the other hand, are the only nuts that contain a significant amount of alpha-linolenic acid, the only type of omega-3 fat that you'll find in plant-based food.

While you're chomping on walnuts, I also want you to consider adding ground flaxseed to your food, which also provides omega-3s, plus 4 grams of fiber per tablespoon. Although technically not a nut, flaxseed has a nutty flavor, so you can add some to your meat or beans, spoon it over cereal, or add a tablespoon to a smoothie.

One caveat, before you go all nutty: Nuts are high in calories, and smoked and salted nuts don't make the cut here because of their high sodium content. High sodium can lead to high blood pressure.

Yogurt and Other Dairy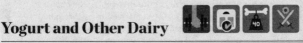

8-HOUR POWERS: Build strong bones, fire up weight loss
SECRET WEAPONS: Calcium, vitamins A and B_{12}, riboflavin, phosphorus, potassium
FIGHTS AGAINST: Osteoporosis, obesity, high blood pressure, cancer
SIDEKICKS: Fat-free or low-fat milk, cheese, and cottage cheese
IMPOSTERS: Whole milk, ice cream, frozen yogurt, sugary fruit-on-the bottom yogurts

Dairy is nutrition's version of a typecast actor. It gets so much attention for one thing it does well—strengthening bones—that it gets little or no attention for all the other stuff it does well. It's about time for dairy to accept a breakout role as a vehicle for weight loss. Just take a look at the mounting evidence: A University of Tennessee study found that dieters who consumed between 1,200 and 1,300 milligrams of calcium a day lost nearly twice as much weight as dieters consuming less calcium. In a Purdue University study of 54 people, those who took in 1,000 milligrams of calcium a day (about 3 cups of fat-free milk) gained less weight over 2 years than those with low-calcium diets.

50 Shades of Whey

Discover a fat-burning superfood

Powdered whey, an animal protein derived from dairy products, packs a fitness and weight-loss wallop. You'll find it in the health-food or supplement section of your supermarket—usually in the sorts of giant plastic bottles that weightlifters like to carry around. There's a reason why they go for the stuff—and why you should too, even if amassing Herculean muscles isn't on your to-do list.

Whey is a high-quality protein packed with essential amino acids that build muscle and burn fat. Because muscle tissue is more metabolically active than fat is, whey can actually trigger your body to burn more calories throughout the day. And you don't need to sip a fancy protein drink with one hand while you curl dumbbells with another: A 2011 study published in the *Journal of Nutrition* showed that, as long as you consume whey within 24 hours of exercise, it will help you tone and sculpt your physique.

But the benefits don't end at vanity. Whey protein is a good source of cysteine, which your body uses to build a cancer–fighting antioxidant called glutathione. Adding just a small amount to your diet may increase glutathione levels in your body by up to 60 percent. And by reducing your risk of obesity, whey is providing you with even greater cancer-fighting protection.

There are two easy ways to add whey to your diet. First, pick up a container of the powdered stuff at your local drug store chain or health food store. Blend a few tablespoons into a smoothie (see Chapter 8 for recipes). The second easy way: Pick up the phone and call your favorite Italian restaurant. Ricotta cheese—a staple in Italian cooking—is made from whey, the liquid drained off during the making of cheeses like mozzarella. Book a table at Giuseppi's, and order up some anticancer lasagna (with ricotta) tonight!

Some researchers think that calcium probably prevents weight gain by increasing the breakdown of body fat and hampering its formation. Another theory, based on a new study in the *British Journal of Nutrition*, suggests that the brain may detect when the body isn't getting enough calcium and signal your body to eat more food to make up for the deficit. So, making sure you consume enough calcium can play an important role in your weight-loss efforts. Chow down on low-fat yogurt, cheeses, and other dairy products every day. But I recommend milk as your major source of calcium for one primary reason: volume. Liquids can take up valuable room in your stomach and send the signal to your brain that you're full. Adding in a sprinkle of chocolate powder can also help curb sweet cravings while still providing nutritional power.

Beans, Peanuts, and Other Legumes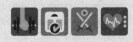

8-HOUR POWERS: Boost testosterone (good for your sex drive as well, ladies!), build muscle, help burn fat, regulate digestion
SECRET WEAPONS: Fiber, protein, iron, folate, monounsaturated fat, vitamin E, niacin, magnesium
FIGHTS AGAINST: Obesity, muscle loss, wrinkles, cardiovascular disease, colon cancer, heart disease, high blood pressure
SIDEKICKS: Lentils, peas, bean dips, hummus, edamame, plus peanut, cashew, and almond butters
IMPOSTERS: Refried beans, which are high in saturated fats; baked beans, which are high in sugar; mass-produced sugary and trans-fatty peanut butters

---

Most of us can trace our resistance to beans to some unfortunately timed intestinal upheaval (third-grade math class, a first date gone awry). But beans are, as the song says, good for your heart; the more you eat them, the more you'll be able to control your hunger. Black, lima, pinto, garbanzo—you pick the bean. You're guaranteed to have a low-calorie food packed with protein, fiber, and iron—ingredients crucial for building muscle and losing weight. Beans serve as one of the key members of the 8-Hour Powerfood team because of all their nutritional power. In fact, if you can swap in a bean-heavy dish for a meat-heavy dish a couple of times per week, you'll be subtracting a lot of saturated fat from your diet and adding high amounts of fiber.

Studies show that regular bean eaters weigh less than those who don't eat beans. Check out some other superpowers of specific beans:

THE MUSCLE BUILDER: SOYBEANS. Technically a legume, soybeans are one of the only common plant foods that contains complete protein, making them terrific muscle-building meat substitutes for vegetarians.

THE CANCER KILLER: LENTILS. Women who eat lentils frequently have a lower risk of developing breast cancer, says a study in the *International Journal of Cancer*. Other studies show that lentils may protect against prostate and colorectal cancers.

THE DIABETES DESTROYER: GARBANZO BEANS. Also known as chickpeas, garbanzos are high in fiber, which helps stabilize blood sugar, lowering the risk of type 2 diabetes (ditto, the 8-Hour Diet). Add them to salads and soups. Chickpeas (mashed) are the main ingredient in hummus, a garlicky bean spread that's terrific on crackers or as a healthier substitute for mayonnaise on sandwiches.

THE ANTIAGING AGENT: RED KIDNEY BEANS. This chili staple contains more antioxidants and omega-3s than any of its bean brethren, plus thiamine, which may be protective against Alzheimer's disease (ditto, the 8-Hour Diet).

THE HEART HEALER: NAVY BEANS. They have the most cholesterol-clobbering fiber of any bean at 10.5 grams per 100-gram serving, plus tons of potassium.

THE BRAIN BOOSTER: BLACK BEANS. Great in breakfast burritos, black beans are full of anthocyanins, compounds that have been shown to improve brain function (ditto . . . aw, you know).

I'll admit that I'm trying to do a sell job on beans. They're an extraordinarily important, health-boosting food, and many of us still leave them on the plate. Contrast that with a food that is synonymous with Mom, Saturday afternoon lunch, and our national pastime: Mr. Peanut, come on down (and leave the Cracker Jacks behind)! He too is part of your 8-Hour power nexus.

Yes, the most common way we dine on this legendary legume—peanut butter—has its disadvantages: It tends to stick to the roof of your mouth, it's high in calories, and it doesn't go over well when you order peanut butter in four-star restaurants. But it's packed with those heart-healthy monounsaturated fats that can increase your body's production of testosterone, which can help your muscles grow and your fat melt. It's also a key sex-drive booster in both men and women, which is one reason Mr. Peanut is so sexy.

But, back to the health benefits. In one 18-month experiment, people who integrated peanut butter into their diet maintained weight loss better than those on low-fat plans. A recent study from the University of Illinois showed that diners who had monounsaturated fats before a meal (in this case, it was olive oil) ate 25 percent fewer calories during that meal than those who didn't. Practically speaking, peanut butter also works because it's a quick and versatile snack (keep a small jar handy at work to fend off hunger pangs). And it tastes great. Since a diet that includes an indulgence like peanut butter doesn't leave you feeling deprived, it's easier to follow and won't make you fall prey to a craving for, say, glazed doughnuts or potato chips. Use PB on an apple, on the go, or to add flavor to potentially bland smoothies.

For variety, try almond butter as a replacement for peanut butter on celery sticks or with whole-fruit or jelly on whole-wheat bread. Nutrition-wise, almond butter offers a bit more fiber and vitamin E and about the same amount of fat and calories as peanut butter.

While we're on the topic of fat and calories, remember these two caveats: You shouldn't gorge on nut butters because of their high fat content; limit yourself to about 3 tablespoons per day. And you should stock up on all-natural peanut butter, not the mass-produced brands that have added sugar and too much salt.

The Health Boosters

A lot of us grew up with an aversion to fruits and vegetables, sometimes caused by doting moms who boiled canned greens into pulp and then insisted that by not eating them, we were somehow responsible for kids in China not having enough rice. Today, you've got two ways to prove your mom wrong: first, by showing her how really delicious fresh produce can be, if you know how to choose and prepare it; and second, by showing her the medal totals from the last two Summer Olympics. (Hey, somebody has been getting enough rice.)

But even if Mom beat all the flavor and texture out of vegetables on the way to the table and served fruit under a gloppy coat of sugar syrup, she was right about one thing: the nutritional value of produce. Nothing quite matches the low-calorie, high-nutrient, high-belly-filling qualities of vegetables. If you incorporate them into your 8-Hour feeding plan, you'll max out on the health and weight-loss benefits, and you can do so while indulging in deliciousness as well.

Raspberries and Other Berries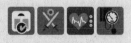

8-HOUR POWERS: Protect your heart; enhance eyesight; improve balance, coordination, and short-term memory; prevent cravings

SECRET WEAPONS: Antioxidants, fiber, vitamin C, tannins (cranberries)

FIGHTS AGAINST: Heart disease, cancer, obesity

SIDEKICKS: The frozen-berry smorgasbord in the freezer case

IMPOSTERS: Jellies, most of which eliminate fiber and add sugar

Depending on your taste, any berry will do (except Crunch Berries). I like raspberries as much for their nutrition as for their taste. They carry powerful levels of antioxidants, and the berry's flavonoids may also help your eyesight, balance, coordination, and short-term memory. One cup of raspberries packs 6 grams of fiber and more than half of your daily requirement of vitamin C.

Blueberries are also loaded with the soluble fiber that, like oatmeal, keeps you fuller longer. In fact, they're one of the most healthful foods you can eat. Blueberries beat out 39 other fruits and vegetables in the antioxidant power ratings. (One study also found that rats that ate blueberries were more coordinated and smarter than rats that didn't.) Psst: Frozen blueberries are just as good for you as the fresh ones.

Strawberries contain another valuable form of fiber called pectin (as do grapefruits, apples, peaches, and oranges). In a study from the *Journal of the American College of Nutrition*, subjects drank plain orange juice or juice spiked with pectin. The people who drank the loaded juice felt fuller after drinking it than those who got the juice without pectin. The difference lasted for an impressive 4 hours.

And you've no doubt heard of the heart-health benefits of swallowing a baby aspirin every day. Well, berries present a much more pleasurable way of taking your medicine. Raspberries, strawberries, and blueberries are all packed with the salicylic acid, the same heart-disease fighter found in aspirin.

Apples, Oranges, and Other Fruits

8-HOUR POWERS: Fill your belly, fight cancer

SECRET WEAPONS: Antioxidants, fiber, vitamin C

FIGHTS AGAINST: Heart disease, cancer, obesity, scurvy (arrrrrh, matey!)

SIDEKICKS: Watermelon, cantaloupe, avocado, tomato

IMPOSTERS: Fruit juices, which concentrate sugar and strip out fiber; many of them have more calories than Coke.

Aside from the clock you'll now be eating by, the most effective weight-loss tool in your home just might be the fruit bowl. If you keep it filled with crisp apples, ripening peaches and plums, citrus, and fuzzy kiwi fruit, you'll have handy snacks that serve you nutritionally and stick with you to curb your appetite. If you can retrain your noshing instinct to end at the fruit bowl, you might quite literally never be hungry again.

Just like strawberries, apples—known as "nature's toothbrush"—are rich in pectin fiber. A recent Penn State study demonstrated the fiber's power as a weight-loss tool: People who ate an apple 15 minutes before lunch ended up consuming 187 fewer calories during the meal than those who didn't snack beforehand. And all that apple chomping isn't just a good workout for your jaw; it tricks your brain into thinking you're eating more than you really are, say the researchers.

And consider the grapefruit. In a study of 100 obese people at the Scripps Clinic in California, those who ate half a grapefruit with each meal lost an average of 3.6 pounds over the course of 12 weeks. Many lost more than 10 pounds. The study's control group, in contrast, lost a paltry half pound. But here's something even better: Those who ate grapefruit also exhibited a decrease in insulin levels, indicating that their bodies had improved upon the ability to metabolize sugar. It could be the optimal fast-breaking fruit, especially because it will give you a massive dose of lycopene—the cancer-preventing antioxidant found most commonly in tomatoes.

And yes, tomatoes—just like their MVP salad companion, the avocado—are fruits, even though it's hard to think of them that way. Summertime, when both of them are at their peak in flavor and nutritional impact, is the healthiest eating time of the year simply because these superstars are in midseason form. Toss them into everything you eat— they're that good for you.

Spinach and Other Green Vegetables

8-HOUR POWERS: Neutralize free radicals, which are molecules that accelerate the aging process
SECRET WEAPONS: Vitamins including A, C, and K; folate; minerals including calcium and magnesium; fiber; beta-carotene
FIGHTS AGAINST: Cancer, heart disease, stroke, obesity, osteoporosis
SIDEKICKS: Cruciferous vegetables such as broccoli; green, yellow, red, and orange vegetables such as asparagus, peppers, and yellow beans
IMPOSTERS: None, as long as you don't fry them or smother them in fatty cheeses

I like spinach in particular because it's such an efficient vegetable: One serving supplies nearly a full day's worth of vitamin A and half of your vitamin C. It's also loaded with folate—a vitamin that protects against heart disease, stroke, and colon cancer.

To incorporate it into your 8-Hour food plan, you can take the fresh stuff and use it as lettuce on a sandwich, or try stir-frying it with a little chopped garlic and olive oil. You can always guarantee that you have spinach handy by stocking up on the frozen chopped variety. Packed right after picking, the frozen stuff is full of the essential nutrients. And frozen spinach conveniently boosts the nutritional value of eggs, soups, and sauces.

Another potent power vegetable is broccoli. It's high in fiber and more densely packed with vitamins and minerals than almost any other food. For instance, it contains nearly 90 percent of the vitamin C of fresh orange juice and almost half as much calcium as milk. It is also a powerful defender against diseases like cancer because it increases the enzymes that help detoxify carcinogens. Tip: With broccoli, you can skip the stalks. The florets have three times as much beta-carotene as the stems, and they're also a great source of other antioxidants. If you hate vegetables, you can learn to hide them but still reap the benefits. Try pureeing them and adding them to marinara sauce or chili. The more you chop and puree vegetables, the more invisible they become and the easier it is for your body to absorb them. With broccoli, sauté it in garlic and olive oil and douse it with hot sauce.

Moving on now to the leafy greens, each of which has a specific superpower you should take advantage of. It's kind of like the *Avengers* on your plate: If you need help, they'll be there (without the leotard).

THE BONE BUILDER: ARUGULA. One cup has 10 percent of the bone-building mineral found in a glass of whole milk and 100 percent less saturated fat. There's also some magnesium in every bite, for more protection against osteoporosis.

THE BREATH PROTECTOR: WATERCRESS. It's a pepper-flavored HEPA filter for your body. Watercress contains phytochemicals that may prevent cigarette smoke and other airborne pollutants from causing lung cancer.

THE ANTIAGING AGENT: BOK CHOY. Think of it as a cabbage-flavored multivitamin. A bowl of bok choy has 23 percent of your daily requirement of vitamin A and a third of your vitamin C, along with three tongue-twisting, cancer-fighting, age-reducing phytochemicals: flavonoids, isothiocyanates, and dithiolethione.

THE SIGHT SHARPENER: SPINACH. Spinach is a top source of lutein and zeaxanthin, two powerful antioxidants that protect your vision from the ravages of old age. A Tufts University study found that frequent spinach eaters had a 43 percent lower risk of age-related macular degeneration.

THE CANCER KILLER: ROMAINE. This celery-flavored green is one of the best vegetable sources of beta-carotene—712 micrograms per cup. A University of Illinois study showed that high levels of beta-carotene inhibited the growth of prostate cancer cells by 50 percent.

THE HEART HEALER: ENDIVE. It's slightly bitter and a little crisp, and it offers twice the fiber of iceberg lettuce. A cup of endive also provides almost 20 percent of your daily requirement of folate. People who don't consume enough of this essential B vitamin may have a 50 percent greater risk of developing heart disease.

THE BRAIN BOOSTER: MUSTARD GREENS. These spicy, crunchy greens are packed with the amino acid tyrosine. In a recent US military study, researchers found that eating a tyrosine-rich meal an hour before taking a test helped soldiers significantly improve both their memories and their concentration. So if at first you don't succeed, tyrosine, tyrosine again.

Whole-Grain Breads and Cereals, including Oatmeal

8-HOUR POWERS: Prevent your body from storing fat
SECRET WEAPONS: Fiber, protein, thiamin, riboflavin, niacin, pyridoxine, vitamin E, magnesium, zinc, potassium, iron, calcium
FIGHTS AGAINST: Obesity, cancer, high blood pressure, heart disease
SIDEKICKS: Brown rice, whole-wheat pretzels, whole-wheat pastas
IMPOSTERS: Processed bakery products like white bread, bagels, and doughnuts; breads labeled wheat instead of whole wheat

There's only so long a person can survive on an all-protein diet or an all-salad diet or an all-anything diet. You will crave carbohydrates because your body needs carbohydrates. The key is to eat the ones that have been the least processed—carbs that still have all their heart-healthy, belly-busting fiber intact.

Grains such as wheat, corn, oats, barley, and rye are seeds that come from grasses, and they're broken into three parts—the germ, the bran, and the endosperm. Think of a kernel of corn. The biggest part of the kernel—the part that blows up when you make popcorn—is the endosperm. Nutritionally it's pretty much a big dud. It contains starch, a little protein, and some B vitamins.

Pick a Peck of Produce

Finding the snappiest fruits and vegetables

AVOCADOS. Feel for firm flesh. Toss back avocados with sunken, mushy spots. They should not rattle when shaken; that's a sign the pit has pulled away from the dried-out flesh.

BERRIES. Before you buy raspberries or strawberries, flip the carton over. You're looking for nature's expiration date: juice stains.

CANTALOUPE. Don't knock on a melon to check its ripeness; slap it instead. You're listening for a hollow ring, not a dull thud or an inhuman scream.

CORN ON THE COB. The sweetest ears are slightly immature, with kernels that don't go all the way to the end of the cob. Toss 'em, husks and all, onto a medium-hot grill. Cook for 10 minutes, then peel back all but the last layer of husk. Grill 5 more minutes for that just-smoked flavor.

KALE. The smaller the leaves, the more tender the kale. Avoid wilted foliage with discolored spots. You want moist leaves with a dark blue-green color.

PEACHES. Look for well-colored fruit with no green spots. The flesh should yield slightly when lightly pressed and should have a fragrant aroma. (Fragrant like a peach, not fragrant like your cousin Freddy.)

TOMATOES. Look for tomatoes that are firm and heavy for their size. They should have a sweet tomato aroma. If you generally don't like tomatoes, try the yellow kind; they tend to have a sweeter, less acidic flavor than red varieties.

WATERMELON. Forget color, shape, or size: Watermelons are best judged by weight. The heavier a melon is, the more water it contains, and water is what helps give a melon its flavor.

The germ is the smallest part of the grain; in the corn kernel, it's that little white seedlike thing. But while it's small, it packs the most nutritional power. It contains protein, oils, and the B vitamins thiamin, riboflavin, niacin, and pyridoxine. It also has vitamin E and the minerals magnesium, zinc, potassium, and iron.

The bran is the third part of the grain and the part where all the fiber is stored. It's a coating around the endosperm that contains B vitamins, zinc, calcium, potassium, magnesium, and other minerals.

So what's the point of this little botany lesson? Well, get this: When food manufacturers process and refine grains, guess which two parts get tossed out? Yup, the bran, where all the fiber and minerals are, and the germ, where all the protein and vitamins are. And what they keep—the nutritionally bankrupt endosperm (that is, starch)—is made into pasta, bagels, white bread, white rice, and just about every other wheat product and baked good you'll find.

Crazy, right?

But if you eat products made with all the parts of the grain—whole-grain bread and pasta, long-grain rice—you get all the nutrition that food manufacturers are otherwise trying to strip away.

Whole-grain carbohydrates can play an important role in a healthy lifestyle. In an 11-year study of 16,000 middle-age people, researchers at the University of Minnesota found that consuming three daily servings of whole grains can reduce a person's mortality risk over the course of a decade by 23 percent. (Tell that to your buddy who's eating low carb.) Whole-grain bread keeps insulin levels low, which keeps you from storing fat. In this diet, it's especially versatile because it'll supplement any kind of meal with little prep time. Whole-wheat toast for brunch, sandwiches for lunch, with a dab of peanut butter for a snack. Don't believe the hype. Carbs—the right kind of carbs—are good for you.

Warning: Food manufacturers are very sneaky. Sometimes, after refining away all the vitamins, fiber, and minerals from wheat, they'll add molasses to the bread, turning it brown, and put it on the grocery shelf with a label that says wheat bread. It's a trick! Truly nutritious breads and other products will say whole wheat or whole grain. Don't be fooled.

Oatmeal is the Michael Bloomberg of your pantry: Kind

of bland on the surface, but bursting with big ideas for your future. Rich in fiber and nutrients, it can propel you through sluggish mornings, or you can eat it a couple of hours before a workout to feel fully energized by the time you hit the weights. Swap it in for your late-night snack to avoid a binge. I recommend instant oatmeal for its convenience. But I want you to buy the unsweetened, flavor-free variety and use other Powerfoods such as milk, berries, and cinnamon to enhance the taste. Flavored oatmeal packets often come loaded with sugar calories.

Oatmeal contains soluble fiber, meaning that it attracts fluid and stays in your stomach longer than insoluble fiber (like vegetables). Soluble fiber is thought to reduce blood cholesterol by binding with digestive acids made from cholesterol and sending them out of your body. When this happens, your liver has to pull cholesterol from your blood to make more digestive acids, and your bad cholesterol levels drop.

Trust me: You need more fiber, both soluble and insoluble. Doctors recommend we eat between 25 and 35 grams of fiber per day, but most of us consume half that. Fiber is like a bouncer for your body, kicking out troublemakers and showing them the door. It protects you from heart disease. It protects you from colon cancer by sweeping carcinogens out of the intestines quickly.

A Penn State study also showed that oatmeal sustains your blood sugar levels longer than many other foods, which keeps your insulin levels stable and ensures you won't be ravenous for the few hours that follow. That's good, because spikes in the production of insulin slow your metabolism and send a signal to the body that it's time to start storing fat. Since oatmeal breaks down slowly in the stomach, it causes less of a spike in insulin levels than foods like bagels. Include it in a smoothie or as your breakfast.

Another cool fact about oatmeal: Preliminary studies indicate that oatmeal raises the levels of free testosterone in your body, enhancing your body's ability to build muscle and burn fat and boosting your sex drive.

The Forgotten Grain

Although it's not yet common in America's kitchens, quinoa (pronounced KEEN-wa) boasts a stronger distribution of nutrients than any grain you'll ever stick a fork into. It has more fiber and nearly twice as much protein as brown rice, and the proteins in it consist of a near-perfect blend of amino acids, the body's building blocks for tissue repair and muscle generation. And get this: All that protein and fiber—in conjunction with a handful of healthy fats and a comparatively small dose of carbohydrates—help ensure a low impact on your blood sugar. That's great news for prediabetics and anyone watching their weight. So what's the trade-off? There is none. Quinoa's mild and nutty taste is easy to handle even for picky eaters, and it cooks just like rice, ready in about 15 minutes. Take that, Uncle Ben.

Also, I want you to consider adding ground flaxseed to your food. I said this before and it bears repeating. One tablespoon contains only 60 calories, but it packs in omega-3 fatty acids and has nearly 4 grams of fiber. Sprinkle it into a lot of different recipes, add some to your oatmeal, spoon it over cereal, or add a tablespoon to a smoothie.

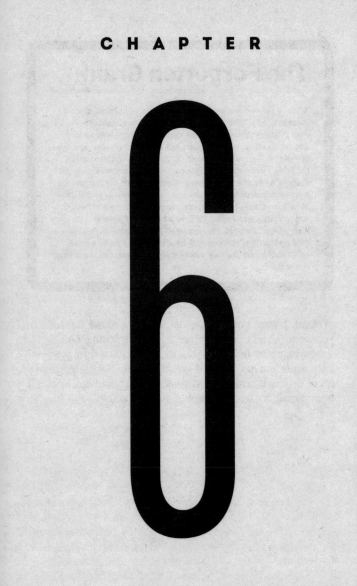

THE 8-HOUR DIET

The 8-Hour Sample Eating Plan

A typical day on a most atypical diet plan

B y now, you must be wondering: What's the catch?

A diet in which you can eat anything you want in whatever quantity you want? One that requires just 8 minutes of exercise a day? One that's proven to strip off up to 2 pounds a day? It can't be that simple!

Oh, but it is. The 8-Hour Diet is so simple, even a caveman could do it (assuming he was willing to give up the Paleo Diet).

Now, I don't blame you for being skeptical. If I had a nickel in my pocket for every diet book that has crossed my desk in the past 20 years, I'd have, well, very heavy pants. But despite the hundreds of weight-loss plans I've seen at *Men's Health*, in truth, they all fall into a handful of familiar categories.

There are the diets that say, "Let them eat numbers!" That is, they assign numerical values to foods or create exact ratios of what should be eaten at every meal, so your calculator winds up working as hard as you are. Weight Watchers is a perfect example—a lot more perfect than its competitors, quite frankly, especially with its recently revamped points system. And if you can hang with the arithmetic, great. But when I'm ready to eat, there are only three kinds of numbers I care about: numbers that get me a reservation, numbers that tell me how long the microwave should run, and numbers that make pizza magically appear on my doorstep. I'm Hungry Man, not Rain Man!

There are the diets that say, "Let them eat grapefruit!" Or cabbage soup. Or bananas. Or Subway sandwiches. Or so much beef that mad cow disease becomes a little too personal. The common denominator here: tricking you into believing that if you fill up on one food, it will crowd out all the others. Which it will—until, like a drunken frat boy, you get caught raiding the fridge with your nutritional pants down. Staying faithful to family, friends, and countrymen? Yes. Having a monogamous relationship with a sandwich shop? That's just not going to work. (Besides, I heard the sandwich shop was seeing other people.)

There are diets that say, "Don't let them eat _____!" No carbs! No sugar! No beer! Dr. Atkins was the founding father of this movement, banishing all carbohydrates—even fruits and vegetables—in favor of meat and more meat. Which does in fact work, until your cravings build to the point where you're chasing the Wonder Bread truck down the street, sniffing fumes. Man cannot live on chicken wings alone; eventually, you need a celery stick.

There are diets that say, "Let them eat only stuff they've cooked in their own kitchens!" I could also call this the Unemployed Celebrity Chef Diet, as there are plenty of cookbooks out there by stars who fancy themselves nutrition experts all of a sudden. Now eat this? Now get real! Cooking at home is usually healthier, yes. But if you have time to cook yourself breakfast, lunch, and dinner 7 days a week, chances are you're just a bit less busy than you should be in other aspects of your life.

And finally, there are diets that say, "Eat what we send you in this very expensive box every night, because fat former sports stars (or their coaches) eat it!" Home delivery is to lifelong nutrition what a stick of dynamite is to fishing. It'll deliver you a meal all right, but very, very expensively. And over time, it's a plan that's just not sustainable.

So why are there still so many schemes and gimmicks out there? Because just about any diet plan will work, at least for a little while. When you have to cut out types or amounts of food, you're participating in a form of calorie restriction. It "works" in two ways. First: If you eat only cabbage soup, Subway sandwiches, or bacon for breakfast, lunch, and dinner, there is only so much room for other indulgences in your life. Second: After about 3 weeks, you'll get so sick of coldcut combos and teenagers wearing plastic gloves, you won't be able to choke down one more sandwich. And then you'll go running back into the arms of the dysfunctional food relationships that made you feel so bad in the first place.

The only way to really make a new diet work is by incorporating healthy new habits that become second nature to you. It's not a new diet, in fact—it's a new way of living. You form eating habits you can stick with forever and that don't require you to stop scratching culinary itches you've had your whole life.

Building these habits are what the 8-Hour Diet is all about. Notice that we're restricting eating times, not specific foods. So you won't crave any favorite food; you'll simply eat it at the right time. In fact, you'll be eating so much that you'll easily fit in all of the 8-Hour Powerfoods and be able to say—probably even before dinner—"I ate my 8!"

It's simple, and you'll soon reach the point where you can stick with it without even thinking. Eat now, fast later can become the equivalent of breathe in, breathe out. And so it can go for the rest of your long and healthy lifetime.

That's what this chapter is for: to show you the feast, the better to help you embrace the fast that wraps around it.

To illustrate what a day of eating on the 8-Hour Diet looks like, I've enlisted my friend Debbie, who is in fact an actual friend who follows this actual routine. Do you have to arrange your life exactly like Debbie has? Absolutely not. Whether you're a nine-to-fiver or a graveyard shifter or a lineman for the county, you can pick up the plan at whatever hour works for you. Here's how Debbie does it.

7:00 AM Popping out of bed bright and early to her alarm (okay, after three consecutive snooze-button bashings), Debbie sleepwalks into the kitchen for coffee. After a full cup of joe and a sobering first look at the world on her tablet, she makes her way to the living room for her ridiculously efficient 8 minutes of exercise. (Yes, that's right—8 minutes is all you need.) Deb doesn't like to work too hard in the morning—she'll just pick and choose from the 20 different 8-minute workouts in Chapter 10, doing just enough to make her heart pump, her muscles vibrate, and—most important—her body metabolize the extra glucose stored in her liver, so she can quickly enter the fat-burning zone. She usually washes down her workout with a zero-calorie drink like SmartWater.

8:30 AM After Deb showers and dresses, it's back to the kitchen to blend up 2 cups of frozen berries, some frozen mango, a few big spoonfuls of Greek yogurt, a splash of OJ, and whiz! Smoothie. But she's not going to drink it now. She pours part of it into an insulated thermos (essential for maintaining both the temperature and texture of her morning creation), stashes the remainder in the fridge for her husband, feeds the cat (because he always forgets to), grabs coffee, and sets her coordinates for work.

10:30 AM While coworkers are milling about, nibbling on Egg McMuffins or standing in line at the company cafeteria, Debbie burns quickly through the battery of e-mails that came in overnight, then catches up on some nagging problems left over from the day before. By 10, she's already well ahead of the game. At last her appetite begins to rouse from its slumber. Luckily, that thermos has everything she needs: The fruit packs fiber, the juice provides a big dose of calcium and vitamin C, and the Greek yogurt gives her a dollop of healthy fat and twice as much protein as regular yogurt. Debbie can down it all in a few spirited gulps or savor the smoothie throughout the morning. 8-Hour Powerfood daily total: 3.

11:30 AM With the day's second meeting out of the way and lunchtime approaching, Deb's increasingly lean belly starts to rumble. It needs something solid. There's a deli around the corner, but to save time, Deb usually stashes a snack—say, a batch of hummus and a bag of pitas—in the fridge in the break room on Monday mornings. Now on her second snack in just over an hour, she's locked in and still plowing through e-mails. 8 Hour Powerfood daily total: 4.

1:00 PM On light days, Deb can take time to treat herself to a leisurely lunch with friends at a local Mexican joint. But there aren't a lot of light days, so she calls up the deli and has them deliver a roast turkey sandwich on whole wheat with cheese, guacamole, and a bit of crispy bacon. People at the office have to wonder—how can she eat so much and still stay so slim? There's nothing to hide here: lean protein, a good dose of fiber, plenty of healthy fat from the avocado. This is exactly what Deb's body needs right now. (And that bacon? One of the most delicious 70-calorie investments you can make.) 8-Hour Powerfood daily total: 7.

3:00 PM Did a hypnotist sweep through the office? Most of the cubicle dwellers have hit their midafternoon slump and are plodding like zombies to the coffee machine or to top off the tank with a Danish. But the increased energy most people see on the 8-Hour Diet keeps Debbie's mind humming while everyone else's is numbing. And there's no reason for Debbie not to snack—she can eat what she wants, as much as she wants, so she reaches under her desk for some chips and salsa—the peppers and tomatoes will help her check off another 8-Hour Powerfood. 8 Hour Powerfood daily total: 8. Ding ding ding! It's only midafternoon, and already Deb ate her 8!

4:00 PM Finally, a break in the action. Deb steps out for a late-afternoon pick-me-up—a tall Americano, just what she needs. And the benefit goes well beyond the jolt of caffeine: According to research from the University of Scranton in Pennsylvania, coffee is the number one source of antioxidants in the American diet. An Americano, espresso diluted with hot water, is the superstar of the modern coffee bar, since, like black coffee, it's essentially a calorie-free drink. But because she's indulging for these 8 hours, Deb pours in a generous glunk of whole milk; it adds just 40 calories, but what a great 40 they are. Why not grab a piece of dark chocolate or a package of almonds as well?

6:00 PM Arriving home, Deb doesn't hesitate. There's so much delicious food to choose from. Perhaps tonight she and her husband will talk about their day over a juicy, freshly ground sirloin burger smothered in caramelized onions. No, this isn't dinner at the local watering hole, and it isn't cheating. This is her creation, made in a matter of minutes on her stove top (see the recipe on page 161). This isn't a diet that trades butter for margarine, Cheddar for cottage cheese, steak for alfalfa sprouts. These recipes are made with real ingredients for people who love to eat. And even though Deb has already hit all her nutritional notes for the day, she tosses a quick green salad on the side for an extra crunchy health kick.

Wait! Where's dessert? Since Deb wants to eat all she can before her 8 hours are up, she follows dinner with a scoop of ice cream covered with warm chocolate sauce and salty peanuts.

8:00 PM Deb and her husband put on a movie (hey, *Modern Family* is a rerun tonight) and let the last few hours of the night slip quietly away. Normally they might be grabbing popcorn or a bowl of cereal right now, but having eaten so much during the day, Deb is happy to settle for a cup of tea with a small cheat–some low-fat milk and a drizzle of honey. And she didn't just eat, she ate well: burgers and bacon, chips and salsa, turkey and guacamole—all the foods she loves. She can rest easy tonight, knowing her body has everything it needs to keep her full and burning calories until tomorrow morning.

The 7-Day Meal Plan

In Chapter 8, we lay out 51 mouthwatering recipes that will keep you sated and burning calories all day long. Here we've put some of those into a weeklong plan, so you get a full sense of all the great food that awaits.

SUNDAY

BREAKFAST/BRUNCH: Huevos Rancheros (P. 136)
SNACK #1: cantaloupe and ham
LUNCH: The Ultimate Burger (P. 161)
SNACK #2: oatmeal cookie and a glass of 2% milk
DINNER: Loaded Alfredo with Chicken and Vegetables (P. 164)

MONDAY

BREAKFAST: Papaya Berry smoothie (P. 133)
SNACK #1: pear and slices of Brie
LUNCH: Chicken Salad Sandwich with Curry and Raisins (P. 152)
SNACK #2: cup of tomato soup
DINNER: Shrimp Scampi (P. 177)

TUESDAY

BREAKFAST: Sunrise Sandwich with Turkey, Cheddar & Guacamole (P. 135)
SNACK #1: sliced tomato with fresh mozzarella
LUNCH: Spinach & Ham Quiche (P. 146)
SNACK #2: square of dark chocolate
DINNER: Seared Sirloin with Red Wine Mushrooms (P. 170)

WEDNESDAY

BREAKFAST: The Caffeinated Banana smoothie (P. 131)
SNACK #1: whole wheat toast with peanut butter
LUNCH: Pesto-Tuna Melt (P. 156)
SNACK #2: Triscuits with ham and Swiss
DINNER: Chili-Mango Chicken (P. 174)

THURSDAY

BREAKFAST: Oatmeal with Peanut Butter and Banana (P. 140)
SNACK #1: Greek yogurt with chopped strawberries
LUNCH: Chinese Chicken Salad (P. 147)
SNACK #2: chips and salsa
DINNER: Honey-Mustard Salmon with Roasted Asparagus (P. 165)

FRIDAY

BREAKFAST: Yogurt Parfait
(P. 138)
SNACK #1: pita with hummus
LUNCH: Turkey, Bacon, Guacamole
Sandwich (P. 154)
SNACK #2: almonds and
grapes
DINNER: Super Supreme Pizza
(P. 178)

SATURDAY

BREAKFAST/BRUNCH:
Blueberry Pancakes (P. 144)
SNACK #1: bowl of Cheerios with
sliced banana
LUNCH: Chicken–White Bean Chili
(P. 157)
SNACK #2: chips and guacamole
DINNER: Grilled Fish Tacos with
Mango Salsa (P. 163)

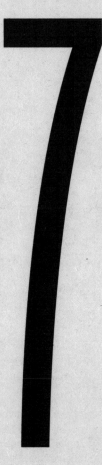

THE 8-HOUR DIET

The 8-Hour Diet Cheat Plan

What to do when your best-laid
8-hour plans are disrupted
by modern life

If life came with a remote control, losing weight would be easy. Need time for the gym? Just hit "pause" on your boss's latest irrational rant and sneak away for a leisurely hour-long workout. Hungry kids in the back seat clamoring for Sonic burgers? Press the "mute" button until you can figure out a healthier eating option. Overdo it on birthday cake? "Rewind" that slice into a half portion.

But in today's world, control is the ultimate luxury—something all of us crave, but few if any of us really have.

Being out of control leads to stress, frustration, and eventually, bad choices. We don't do the things we need to do for ourselves because we can't find the time or the will, or we become overtaxed by all the demands on us and wind up doing dumb things—like skipping greens and doubling down on comfort foods. Either way, the more we feel out of control, the harder it becomes to look good, feel good, and truly enjoy life.

So when faced with the challenge of eating only during a set time period each day, it's easy to conjure scenarios that make it seem impossible. Some meetings need to be breakfast meetings, with an important new client or an even more important old friend. Some dinners need to be late dinners, because the bus was delayed or the first draft of the lasagna came out charred.

And that's when you're planning just for your own meals. Add in kids who need breakfast at 6:30, a hungry spouse who wants dinner at 8, and a gaggle of friends who bring over ice cream at 10—suddenly the 8-Hour Diet looks more like the 18-Hour Diet.

So, no, you're never going to be able to stick to this plan every day. It can't be done, unless you're going into full hermit mode. But that's okay: You don't need to stick to this diet plan every day. In fact, on the 8-Hour Diet, you can cheat as freely as a Mad Man and still lose the weight like crazy. (You devil, Roger!)

The Cheater's Guide to Weight Loss

As you've read in previous chapters, people have lost 10, 20, 30 pounds or more following the 8-Hour Diet a mere 3 days a week! The more you follow it, the better your results—but this is a plan that's designed to conform to your real life.

While I certainly don't follow the eating schedule every day, I know that when I do, I feel sharper, more energetic, and even less hungry than I would otherwise. Indeed, if I've got a serious meeting or a looming deadline, I throw myself into the 8-Hour Diet with abandon, because I know it will sharpen my mind and amp my energy levels.

But I'm as vulnerable to life's curveballs as anyone. So let me walk you through some of the pitfalls I've experienced as I've followed this plan. Many will resonate with you, and you'll see just how easy it is to customize this program to fit your own schedule and needs. And as I walk you through the chaos that is our daily lives, I'll distill eight great rules for cheaters to help you thrive on the 8-Hour Diet.

You see, when I began working on this book, I gathered up a posse of about 2,000 of my closest friends—readers of *Men's Health, Women's Health,* and *Prevention* magazines—and asked them to turn themselves into skinny guinea pigs for the 8-Hour Diet. They responded with incredible enthusiasm, no doubt because they'd never seen "eat what you like" and "lose weight" credibly linked in the same sentence before.

But within just a few days, the emails began coming in: "Do I, um, really have to stick with it every minute of every day? See, my brother-in-law and his wife are coming into town, and we always go to this breakfast buffet . . ."

I knew where they were coming from. The story of my life can pretty much be summed up in four words: "Been there, ate that." It led me down the path of precocious pulchritude as a chubby teenager, and it challenges me now on a weekly schedule that can often veer between a 5 a.m. wakeup call for an appearance on the *Today* show to a late-evening meeting with an author that can drag out over more than one bottle of red wine. Indeed, my "schedule" is no schedule at all.

And while you may not have to face Matt Lauer in the morning, your challenges are just as real—and just as difficult to balance. Like that loyal dieter who wanted to do the right thing and observe the breakfast-buffet tradition with his brother-in-law, we all need to cheat sometimes. Here's how.

CHEATING STRATEGY #1: You don't have to stick with it all the time to succeed.

Early in these pages I described the mechanism whereby your body, during a 16-hour break from eating, quickly burns through the supply of glycogen in the liver and then begins selectively burning body fat.

Awesome, right?

The even better news is that, once you start engaging that mechanism on a regular basis, the health and weight-loss benefits that come with it stick with you, even when you're not doing it all the time. Keep in mind that some of the earliest research done on this approach—the studies that first brought to light the extraordinary health benefits of intermittent fasting—focused on Mormons, who fast *once a month* as a religious observance. A 2008 study published in the *American Journal of Cardiology* found that this practice slashed practitioners' risk of coronary artery disease by 16 percent and significantly reduced their incidence of diabetes, even after adjusting for other healthy habits like abstaining from nicotine and alcohol. So they were doing a version of the 8-Hour Diet, but they were doing it for a total of only 12 days in a year and still enjoying a remarkable health transformation. Devout Muslims observe a daylight fast for the month of Ramadan and return to a typical pattern of eating the other 11 months of the year. They too show health benefits that extend beyond the period of their altered meal plan.

So you can see why this is just about the most flexible diet plan ever created. You shouldn't feel the need to stick to the 8-Hour Diet on a 24/7/365 basis. If you know that Thursday through Sunday will be a forced march of client breakfasts, room-service meals, and bottomless peanut bowls in sports bars, no worries—you'll still be deriving the benefits of the days when you did follow the plan.

The 8-Hour Diet has a kind of momentum of its own, so if you stick with it most of the time, it sticks with you, as well.

If you fall, it catches you.

CHEATING STRATEGY #2: When in doubt, drink.

The one place you don't want to find yourself in the morning is between me and a pot of coffee. If caffeine is a real addiction, then my name is Dave, and I'm a coffeeholic.

But starting the day with coffee or tea, even if you take a little milk or sugar in it, is fine. Caffeine is a mild appetite suppressant, so it helps to see you past the doughnut tray. Plus, it's energizing and helps you concentrate—two of the key mental tricks that keep you from succumbing to any insistent demands sent up from your digestive tract. And coffee and tea are both excellent sources of antioxidants— again, coffee is the number-one source in the American diet. One caveat, though: You're not on the 8-Hour Diet if you're starting your day by drinking down a sugary, high-calorie latte drink. A medium Dunkin' Donuts Coffee Coolatta with Cream is 660 calories and 39 grams of fat. A cup of joe with a little whole milk and sugar is more like 40 calories, and that's an acceptable cheat.

Even if you're not a caffeine lover like me, make sure you start your day with plenty of fluids. Says food researcher David Levitsky, PhD, from Cornell University: "The most important thing about fasting is that you have to have fluids. We can live up to a month without eating calories, but we can't do anything about the fluids. We have to have fluids."

Both hunger and thirst are controlled by a brain region called the hypothalamus. As a result, we often misinterpret thirst as a cry for food. As you contemplate employing Cheat #2, I'd suggest that you turn that common misconception around and drink any time you think you're hungry. Explore some of the new calorie-free beverages out there. For instance, the emergence of Izze sodas on the market, along with SmartWater and every flavor of seltzer under the sun, gives you and me a ton of great-tasting, calorie-free options that weren't available to the Pepsi Generation. In fact, you should learn to indulge in them, savor them, keep them chilled in the fridge and easily at hand. I even keep a refrigerator in my office now, so I can hear that satisfying pssssscccchhhht! whenever thirst tries to trick me into thinking I'm hungry.

CHEATING STRATEGY #3: Occupy your free time.

The best part about the 8-Hour Diet is that you don't have to think about it while you're on it. Instead of deciding whether your meal qualifies as healthy under some sort of arcane point system or zone program, you just look at the clock: Time to eat? Okay, eat—whatever you want, as much as you want. And by adding the 8-Hour Powerfoods into your daily diet, you guarantee maximum nutrition without having to worry about calorie counting or carb-to-fat ratios or other arithmetical gymnastics.

But in weight loss, as in comedy, timing is everything. And even as the leading obesity researchers in the world are telling everyone it's time to cut down on the number of meals, some chain restaurants—that's you, Taco Bell—are trying to convince us that there's something called a "Fourth Meal" that comes sometime between dinner and Jimmy Kimmel. (I'll check the gospels, but I'm pretty sure the Last Supper wasn't followed by the Last Midnight Snack.)

If I had my druthers, I'd just as soon skip breakfast most days, hit the gym at noon, and break my fast between 1 and 2. That extends my eating period to 9 or 10 o'clock, perfect for an on-the-move guy living in a big city. But, given 24 hours notice of that 8 a.m. breakfast with a potential advertiser in *Men's Health* or an even earlier morning-show appearance, I can cheat a new schedule into place. I'll start my 8-Hour feast early and conclude with a late-afternoon megasnack. Same 8-Hour Diet, just a different 8-hour period.

But if I stop eating in the late afternoon, that leaves a lot of hours during the evening in which I might be tempted by those Domino's ads they run on *Monday Night Football*. To make this schedule easier, I'll arrange my evening around a workout, a movie with a friend (sans popcorn), a late writing or work session—anything that will keep my mind active while my jaw is taking a break.

The key goal here: Preserve as much of the 16-hour fast as possible, because that's the mechanism that burns through your glycogen supply and triggers fat burning and the rest of the health effects. Other than that, the timing is entirely up to you. Whatever works best for you is best for you. And that includes the ultimate cheat: just blowing it off for the day. The scientists who study this meal plan don't call it "intermittent fasting" for nothing. The benefits come if you observe it a few times a week, or if those studies of Mormons are to be believed, even once a month. So consider this a flex-time diet: Observe it when you can, ditch it when you can't.

CHEATING STRATEGY #4: Sleep through it.

Look at the reality of what I'm asking you to do on the 8-Hour Diet. You need to string together 16 consecutive hours in which you're putting down the fork and picking up weight-loss and health benefits (same thing). There's hardly any way you can go on this plan without sleeping through most of it, L'il Abner style. The health benefits are yours to keep, simply for not eating while you sleep. It's like checking your bank balance to find that the week's paycheck went in via automatic deposit.

And that also means you've just got two 4-hour periods—one in the morning, one in the evening—to occupy yourself with something other than answering the dinner bell. If I've done my job in writing this book, you'll be armed with literally hundreds of strategies for achieving exactly that.

James B. Johnson, MD, a plastic surgeon at Louisiana State University Medical Center, is one of the most active early researchers into intermittent fasting. He has observed dozens of people on an every-other-day eating plan and has come to know the ins and outs of their challenges and rewards.

Says Dr. Johnson: "It's important to have a procedure to follow when the pressure to eat seems to be too great. Sit down, close your eyes, take four deep breaths, inhale and exhale slowly, visualize enjoying yourself. Get outside, engage someone else, help your children with their homework, or engage in some repetitive simple task."

Another really effective way to maximize your fat burn: Go to bed a little earlier. The sleep/weight loss connection is undeniable (see "Sleep Your Way Younger, Slimmer, and Healthier" on page 27 for evidence that won't put you to sleep, but you'll wish it did). And going to bed earlier will avoid another problem: "If you're in too deprived a caloric state, you secrete a hormone called orexin, which keeps you awake," notes Dr. Johnson. Hitting the hay earlier can short-circuit this issue, but if you need to stay up later, he offers this advice: "Save 100 to 200 calories for bedtime to help you fall asleep."

Is there a better cheat than milk and cookies before bedding down? It's a doctor-approved bedtime snack, after all!

CHEATING STRATEGY #5: Swap in a workout for a meal.

Okay, this "cheating" strategy isn't exactly on the same level as "What happens in Vegas stays in Vegas," I know. But of all the sneaky strategies I employ to remain true to the 8-Hour Diet, exercise may be the most effective. Why?

Three reasons:

Sweat is a perfect distraction. Really, the worst thing you can do during a food craving is: nothing. Idle hands are the Devil Dogs' workshop; left unoccupied, they're soon dropping coins into the vending machine and tearing open the cookie box. For me, a growling stomach is a command to get on my feet and head for the gym. I know that, once I start my workout, my body will overrule my belly until the last repetition is through.

Success is an endorphin rush. I edit fitness articles for a living, so I've completed workouts in all sorts of conditions—including a lot of times when I've started out thinking, "This is going to stink, and I wish I were doing almost anything else." But you know what? At a certain point, an exercise session develops a momentum of its own—equal parts excitement that you're working hard, gladness that now that you've started this will soon be over, plus a little hormonal reward. You've heard of the endorphin rush? It's your body's way of telling you that you're doing the right thing for yourself. Yes, there's satisfaction biting into a fresh scone from Starbucks. But the rush of a workout well concluded makes that pale by comparison.

Movement tells a complaining belly to shut up. When you're exercising, blood is diverted from your internal organs to your muscles and extremities, the parts of the body you're challenging during a workout. It takes a while, postexertion, for blood and energy supplies to return to the gut, where they'd be needed if you were going to digest a meal. Hence, your appetite diminishes while you're in workout-recovery mode.

So, now do you see why I call exercise a cheat? And you don't have to dedicate an hour, a half hour, or even a quarter of an hour to get the benefits. In Chapter 10, I'll show you more than a dozen 8-Minute Workouts that range from a simple power walk to a full-body, no-weights toning routine. In fact, simply by getting up and being active at the first sign of a craving, you're bamboozling your belly while building muscle and endurance.

Who said cheaters never prosper?

CHEATING STRATEGY #6: Use protein as a cheat meal.

- **A JUICY STEAK,** medium rare, with mushrooms in wine sauce
- **BBQ CHICKEN,** with crusty skin, and side dish of baked beans
- **A BACON, EGG,** and cheese burrito, with salsa dribbled on top
- **A HAM STEAK,** with warm pineapple
- **A CHEESEBURGER,** grilled and gooey

What do all of these have in common, aside from being a) awesomely delicious and b) almost always verboten in standard diet plans?

They all provide a healthy dose of protein to use for fuel, which will help your body replace the fat it's burning with the lean, strong muscle that will give your body a top-to-bottom toning.

On the 8-Hour Diet, your body is selectively burning body fat for energy. But it's also going to burn the carbs, fats, and protein you eat during your 8-hour feeding fest. Your goal is to have a little protein left over after your body has burned off all your food intake, so it can maintain and even build more lean muscle.

"If you go on a protein-sufficient but energy-insufficient diet, then you preserve lean tissue and have all these benefits," says Marc Hellerstein, MD, PhD, professor of human nutrition in the Department of Nutritional Sciences and Toxicology at UC Berkeley's College of Natural Resources. In other words, you're signaling your body to selectively burn fat, but you're also letting it know that you want it to preserve, and even build, lean muscle. "This isn't about missing meals, this is about going on a very structured way of eating that convinces the body that you are in a state of caloric insufficiency and that the body needs to respond [by burning fat]."

The perfect time to consume that protein: at your first meal of the day, especially if you did an 8-Minute Workout in the morning. Your body will be craving the building blocks of muscle repair.

CHEATING STRATEGY #7: Invite carbs to dinner!

- **A PLATE OF PASTA,** with grated Parmesan
- **CRUSTY PIZZA,** with plum tomatoes and garlic
- **STIR-FRIED RICE** and vegetables
- **AN EAR OF BUTTER-SLATHERED CORN ON THE COB**—no, two!

All of those meals sound so delicious and carb-tastic, Atkins enthusiasts are weeping into their cottage cheese. But those carb-rich treats will also make it profoundly easier to adhere to, and enjoy, the 8-Hour Diet. A 2011 study in the journal *Obesity* found that consuming most of your carbs at dinner leads to greater weight loss, a reduction in waist size, and a reduction in body fat percentage, compared to spreading your carbs across feedings.

Isn't that awesome? Finally, a diet plan that tells you to eat carbs, instead of just swatting the pasta fork out of your quivering paw.

Interestingly, the *Obesity* study focused on Muslims, who were observing a daylight fast during the month of Ramadan, as I mentioned before. Researchers wanted to see how fasting influenced the body's production of leptin, the "No thanks, I'm full" hormone. And they found that, if you're going to eat carbs, nighttime is the right time.

According to the study: "[Eating carbs at night] induced a single daily insulin secretion in the evening, thus it was predicted that the diet would lead to higher concentrations of leptin starting 6 to 8 hours later, i.e., in the morning and throughout the day. This may lead to enhanced satiety during daylight hours and improve dietary adherence."

After 180 days, more than two-thirds of the group that carbed out in the evening felt their appetites were under control; only 19 percent of dieters who spread out carb consumption through the day said the same. The nighttime carb eaters weren't jonesing for food in the afternoon; a third of the all-day carb eaters were.

Another important thing about this study: Even though the nighttime carb eaters were on a weight-loss program, they didn't have jacked-up hunger levels. Their eating schedule seems to have spared them that.

It's beginning to look like a reliable clock might be more important to weight loss than a reliable scale.

CHEATING STRATEGY #8: Plan your indulgences.

By the time I started writing this book, I'd already read dozens of accounts from people who'd experimented with intermittent fasting. To a man and a woman, they said that during their eating periods, they literally had trouble including all the foods they'd like to eat. In fact, their hunger was so well satisfied, they just couldn't look at another _____ [fill in blank with your favorite food temptation here].

I know exactly what they're talking about. In fact, I tuck into my fast-breaking meal—whatever time of the day it falls in—with gusto. Ditto the other major meal I have during my 8-hour eating time. But there's only so much one stomach can hold, so I make sure I plan my foods carefully.

Hence the steady supply of oranges and dark chocolate almonds—or apples with peanut butter, or parma ham and Swiss cheese—that I make sure to have on hand during my fasting days. No doubt, you have your own list. If not, chef Matt Goulding—my coauthor on the *Eat This, Not That!* and *Cook This, Not That!* books—will be happy to set you up. (Check out the next chapter for your 8-Hour feast.)

But the principle here is simple: If you schedule your indulgences during your 8 hours of eating, as I do, you will be that much less likely to be thinking about them during the 16-hour break you'll take from the food trough. Denial for a lifetime is difficult. Waiting until your next feasting time—not so hard.

BONUS CHEATING STRATEGY: Remember: The next meal is coming soon, and it's going to taste delicious.

Wait: How can I guarantee that your next meal is going to be delicious? I don't have any idea what you're going to eat!

Well, I can guarantee it, and that's not psychic, it's science. According to Donald Leopold, MD, a professor of otolaryngology at the University of Nebraska Medical Center, our tasting organs—your tongue, yes, but your nose, too—evolved largely to distinguish good food from harmful food. So when you slide that first mouthful past your lips, you savor every aspect of it: scent, temperature, texture, flavor. You perceive it as an aesthetic experience, but your body is merely trying to distinguish deliciousness from disaster. Once it declares a food safe, it checks out. (That's why the first time you taste a new gourmet entrée will always be slightly better than the next time.)

Now, project that tasting process out to a full day of eating—from 8 a.m., say, until 11 p.m. It's probably a lot like what you're doing now—a whole lot of mindless eating. Since your body has become so habituated to these foods, the same ones you scarf down day after day, it no longer feels the need to investigate, and register, the flavor as fully.

But when you take a break from eating and come back to the table for the 8-Hour Diet, your senses are heightened. Your taste buds work hard, bringing all the flavors to the fore, and all your meals taste better than ever.

When was the last time anybody said that about dining on a diet?

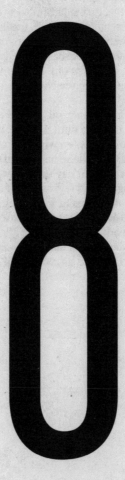

The 8-Minute Recipes

A selection of incredible recipes that incorporate the eight Superfoods and show you how easy it is to eat your 8!

The 8-Hour Diet is so simple and effective because it doesn't in any way restrict the foods you eat, or the amounts you eat. Indeed, nothing's off-limits, and I encourage you to eat until you're satiated. The more satisfied you are with what you're eating, the easier it will be to enjoy your eating time and manage your noneating time.

Which is why hearty, delicious food is so important to the success of this program. If you're going to trek across the desert, there damn well better be a refreshing oasis at the other end. That's why I've asked chef and *New York Times* bestselling author Matt Goulding to put together some of the most delicious, nutritious, satisfying recipes you'll ever taste. And many of them can be prepared in 8 minutes or less.

These recipes pack in nutrients in the form of the 8-Hour Powerfoods, so you'll find it easier than ever to say, "I ate my 8!"

Breakfast/Brunch

While most people following the 8-Hour Diet will choose to skip breakfast, these terrific meals are made to travel, so you can whip them up at home and eat them later in the day. Or linger in bed or over the paper in the morning, then enjoy a hearty weekend brunch. Either way, when it comes time to "break your fast," you'll be doing it with something you love.

SMOOTHIES

The Caffeinated Banana

SUPERFAST SMOOTHIES   With protein, healthy fat, and caffeine, this works perfectly as a start to your day or as a low-cal substitute for a milk shake. As with all of the smoothies in this chapter, a thermos will help you maintain the temperature and texture of a smoothie hours after it's been blended.

- 1 very ripe banana
- ½ cup strong coffee
- ½ cup milk
- 1 Tbsp peanut butter
- 1 Tbsp agave syrup
- 1 cup ice

Combine all ingredients in a blender and mix to your desired consistency.

3 POWER FOODS

1 SERVING

335 CALORIES

12 G FAT

3 G SAT. FAT

38 G SUGARS

4 G FIBER

The Blue Monster

SUPERFAST SMOOTHIES Between the polyphenols in the blueberries and pomegranate and the omega-3s in the flax, we're talking serious brain food.

3 POWER FOODS

1 SERVING

279 CALORIES

5 G FAT

1 G SAT. FAT

41 G SUGARS

6 G FIBER

1	cup blueberries	
½	cup pomegranate or blueberry juice	
½	cup yogurt	
3 or 4	cubes of ice	
1	Tbsp ground flaxseed	

Combine all ingredients in a blender and mix to your desired consistency.

The Orange Crush

SUPERFAST SMOOTHIES All that orange produce means this baby is stuffed full of vision-strengthening, cancer-fighting carotenoids.

3 POWER FOODS

1 SERVING

285 CALORIES

3 G FAT

2 G SAT. FAT

37 G SUGARS

4 G FIBER

¾	cup frozen mango	
½	cup carrot juice	
½	cup orange juice	
½	cup 2% Greek-style yogurt	
1	Tbsp protein powder	
½	cup water	

Combine all ingredients in a blender and mix to your desired consistency.

Papaya Berry

SUPERFAST SMOOTHIES   This is like a liquid mulitvitamin, loaded with vitamins A and C, plus disease-fighting carotenoids and lycopene.

3 POWER FOODS

1 SERVING

¾ cup frozen papaya
¾ cup frozen strawberries
½ cup 1% milk
½ cup orange juice
1 Tbsp fresh mint

Combine all ingredients in a blender and mix to your desired consistency.

188 CALORIES

2 G FAT

1 G SAT. FAT

28 G SUGARS

5 G FIBER

Pineapple Punch

SUPERFAST SMOOTHIES   Like a tropical vacation in a glass. In fact, a shot of rum would turn this into one heck of a healthy cocktail.

2 POWER FOODS

1 SERVING

1 cup frozen pineapple
½ cup 2% Greek-style yogurt
½ cup 1% milk
½ cup orange juice

Combine all ingredients in a blender and mix to your desired consistency.

255 CALORIES

4 G FAT

1 G SAT. FAT

37 G SUGARS

3 G FIBER

The Green Goddess

SUPERFAST SMOOTHIES Fiber and protein combine forces to vanquish any hunger in this untraditional but tasty creation.

4 POWER FOODS

1 SERVING

350 CALORIES

7 G FAT

2 G SAT. FAT

38 G SUGARS

6 G FIBER

- ¼ avocado, peeled and pitted
- 1 ripe banana
- 1 Tbsp honey
- ½ cup 1% milk
- 1 scoop protein powder
- ½ cup ice
- 1 tsp freshly grated ginger (optional)

Combine all ingredients in a blender and mix to your desired consistency.

WEIGHT-LOSS WEAPON

Thomas' Light Multi-Grain English Muffin

Each muffin contains just 100 calories and packs in an astounding 8 grams of fiber—about as much as you'd find in three apples. It provides the perfect base for dozens of handheld breakfasts. Here are a few worth trying.

★ Smoked salmon with tomato and avocado

★ Scrambled eggs with ham, American cheese, and spinach

★ Peanut butter with banana slices and honey

Sunrise Sandwich with Turkey, Cheddar & Guacamole

8 MINUTE MEAL! This sandwich has everything your body needs in the morning hours: protein to jump-start the metabolism, healthy fat and fiber to keep you full until lunch. Make this at home, wrap it in foil, and haul it off to work.

5 POWER FOODS

1 SERVING

380 CALORIES

18 G FAT

5 G SAT. FAT

1,400 MG SODIUM

6 G FIBER

1 tsp canola or olive oil
1 egg
   Salt and black pepper to taste
2 oz smoked turkey breast*
1 slice (¾ oz) American, Cheddar, or pepper Jack cheese
1 thick slice tomato
1 whole-wheat English muffin, split and toasted
1 Tbsp Ultimate Guacamole (page 184) or Wholly Guacamole

*Smoked meat products can be high in sodium. Look for turkey with fewer than 500 milligrams of sodium per serving.

Heat the oil in a small nonstick skillet (see Skillet Secret on page 142) or sauté pan over medium heat until hot. Add the egg and gently fry until the white is set but the yolk is still runny, about 5 minutes. Season with salt and pepper.

Place the turkey on a plate, top with cheese, and microwave for 30 seconds, until the cheese is melted. Place the tomato on the bottom half of the English muffin and season with salt and pepper. Top with the turkey, egg, and guacamole and then with the other muffin half.

Huevos Rancheros

8 MINUTE MEAL! Weekends on the 8-Hour Diet mean time for a long, lazy brunch, and this is just the dish for the job. Smoky black beans, spicy salsa, and a pair of fried eggs will keep you buzzing well into the afternoon.

4 POWER FOODS

4 SERVINGS

375 CALORIES

12 G FAT

3 G SAT. FAT

749 MG SODIUM

10 G FIBER

- 1 can (16 oz) whole peeled tomatoes, with juice
- ½ small onion, chopped
- 1 clove garlic, chopped
- 1 Tbsp chopped chipotle pepper
- ¼ cup chopped fresh cilantro
  Juice of 1 lime
  Salt and black pepper to taste
- 1 can (16 oz) black beans
  Pinch of ground cumin
- 8 eggs
- 8 corn tortillas

Combine the tomatoes, onion, garlic, chipotle, cilantro, and half of the lime juice in a food processor and pulse until well blended but still slightly chunky. Season with salt and pepper.

Mix the black beans, cumin, and remaining lime juice in a bowl; season with salt and pepper. Use the back of a fork to lightly mash up the beans, adding a splash of warm water if necessary.

Coat a large nonstick skillet or sauté pan with nonstick cooking spray and heat over medium heat. Break the eggs into the skillet; cook until the whites have set but the yolks are still loose and runny.

On a separate burner, heat a medium skillet over medium heat and add the tortillas, 2 at a time; cook for 1 minute on each side, until lightly toasted.

To assemble the dish, spread the tortillas with the beans, top with the eggs, and top the eggs with the salsa. Garnish with more cilantro, if you like, and serve immediately.

Waffles with Ham & Eggs

8 MINUTE MEAL! A funky, counterintuitive convergence of salty and sweet flavors, but it works. Trust me.

3 POWER FOODS

4 SERVINGS

- 4 thick slices Canadian bacon or deli ham
- 4 eggs
- 4 frozen whole-grain waffles*
- 2 Tbsp maple syrup
- 4 Tbsp shredded sharp Cheddar cheese
  Salt and black pepper to taste

260 CALORIES

12 G FAT

4 G SAT. FAT

766 MG SODIUM

2 G FIBER

*We like Van's Gourmet Multi-Grain. Each waffle packs 2.5 grams of fiber and just 95 calories.

Heat a nonstick skillet or sauté pan over medium heat. Coat with a bit of olive oil cooking spray and cook the Canadian bacon for a few minutes on each side, until well browned. Remove. Coat the same pan with a bit more spray and cook the eggs (2 at a time, if you must; avoid overcrowding the pan) sunny side up until the whites have set but the yolks are still runny.

In the meantime, toast the waffles. Top each toasted waffle with a slice of meat, a drizzle of maple syrup, a sprinkle of Cheddar, and the warm fried eggs. Season with salt and pepper.

CHANGE IT UP

With a whole-wheat waffle as your base, you can build a slew of sweet and savory open-faced breakfast sandwiches. Try one of these.

★ Peanut butter, sliced banana, sliced almonds, and a drizzle of honey

★ Scrambled eggs, turkey, and guacamole

★ Fresh ricotta or mascarpone cheese, sliced strawberries or figs, and agave syrup

Yogurt Parfait

8 MINUTE MEAL!

Greek yogurt is made with milk that has been skimmed of its watery whey, which gives it an impossibly creamy texture and twice as much protein as standard yogurt. If you haven't already fallen in love with Greek yogurt, this 60-second breakfast will help seal the deal.

1	cup sliced strawberries*
½	cup blueberries (frozen are good, too)*
2	tsp sugar
4 or 5	mint leaves, sliced thinly
1	container (8 oz) low-fat plain Greek-style yogurt (Fage 2% is our favorite)
¼	cup granola

4 POWER FOODS

1 SERVING

358 CALORIES

7 G FAT

4 G SAT. FAT

37 G SUGARS

7 G FIBER

*Any juicy fruit will work well here: raspberries, blackberries, kiwi, mangoes.

Combine the fruit, sugar, and mint in a bowl and allow to sit for 3 to 4 minutes. Spoon half of the yogurt into a bowl or glass, top with half of the fruit and granola, then repeat with the remaining yogurt, fruit, and granola. Pour any accumulated juice from the fruit over the top.

Breakfast Burritos

8 MINUTE MEAL!   This is the kind of power breakfast you will crave after a morning workout session. The whole-wheat tortilla makes it perfectly portable (especially wrapped in foil) but this can just as easily be converted into breakfast tacos by substituting warm corn tortillas.

6 POWER FOODS

4 SERVINGS

468 CALORIES

25 G FAT

9 G SAT. FAT

812 G SUGARS

11 G FIBER

- ½ Tbsp olive oil
- 2 cooked chicken sausage links, diced
- 1 red onion, diced
- 6 eggs, lightly beaten
  Salt and black pepper to taste
  Chopped cilantro
- 4 whole-wheat tortillas (10")
- 1 cup black beans, rinsed, drained, and heated
- ½ cup shredded Cheddar or Jack cheese
- 1 avocado, pitted, peeled, and sliced
- 1 cup of your favorite salsa
  Chopped jalapeños (optional) to taste

Heat the oil in a large skillet or sauté pan over medium heat. Add the sausage and onion; cook for 5 minutes or until lightly browned. Turn the heat to low.

Pour the eggs into the skillet. Cook slowly, constantly stirring with a wooden spoon until the eggs are firm but still moist. Remove from the heat, season with salt and pepper, and stir in the cilantro.

Wrap the tortillas in damp paper towels and heat in the microwave for 45 seconds. (Or heat them individually in a dry pan until warm and lightly toasted.) Divide the eggs, beans, cheese, and avocado among the tortillas. Roll into tight packages and top each burrito with salsa, more cilantro, and jalapeños (if using).

Oatmeal with Peanut Butter and Banana

8 MINUTE MEAL!

Plain oatmeal is boring and flavored packaged oatmeal contains too many funky ingredients and a deluge of added sugars. This recipe solves both problems by combining lightly sweetened home-made oatmeal with the Elvis-approved combination of peanut butter and banana. Make the agave syrup your go-to sweetener; it has the same amount of calories as sugar or honey, but it has a much gentler impact on your blood sugar.

2 POWER FOODS
4 SERVINGS

320 CALORIES
10 G FAT
1 G SAT. FAT
17 G SUGARS
7 G FIBER

4½ cups water
2 cups rolled oats
Pinch of salt
2 bananas, sliced
2 Tbsp peanut butter
¼ cup chopped almonds
2 Tbsp agave syrup

In a medium saucepan, bring the water to a boil. Turn the heat down to low and add the oatmeal and salt. Cook, stirring occasionally, for about 5 minutes, until the oats are tender and have absorbed most of the liquid.

Add the bananas, peanut butter, almonds, and agave syrup and stir to incorporate evenly. If the oatmeal is too thick, add a splash of milk.

CHANGE IT UP

Other ways to dress up a bowl of oatmeal:
★ Diced apples, toasted walnuts, and a pinch of cinnamon
★ Sliced peaches, brown sugar, and chopped pecans (think peach cobbler)
★ Soy sauce, scallions, and a fried egg (trust me—this makes a lot of sense)

Frittata with Arugula and Pepper

8 MINUTE MEAL!   Among the many virtues of a frittata: It takes just minutes to make, packs a perfect balance of lean protein and healthy fat, can be made with dozens of different ingredients, and travels extremely well. Make one on Sunday night and take a wedge to work each day.

4 POWER FOODS

4 SERVINGS

342 CALORIES

24 G FAT

11 G SAT. FAT

752 MG SODIUM

1 G FIBER

½ Tbsp olive oil
¼ cup bottled roasted red peppers, chopped
1 clove garlic, minced
4 cups baby arugula or baby spinach
4 thin slices prosciutto or other good ham, cut into strips
8 eggs, beaten
Salt and black pepper to taste
½ cup crumbled goat cheese or feta

Preheat the broiler. Heat the olive oil in a nonstick, 12" oven-safe skillet over medium-low heat. Add the roasted pepper and garlic and cook for about 1 minute, until the garlic is fragrant but not browned. Stir in the arugula and cook for another 2 minutes or so, until lightly wilted. Add the prosciutto, then pour the eggs over the top. Season the eggs with a good amount of salt and pepper, then dot with the crumbled goat cheese.

Cook on the stovetop for 5 to 6 minutes, until most of the egg has set. Place the pan 6" under the broiler and cook for about 3 minutes, until the rest of the egg has fully set and the top of the frittata has begun to brown. Cool slightly, remove from the pan, and cut into wedges.

CHANGE IT UP

Don't take the ingredients in this recipe too literally; rather, learn the basic technique, then play around with the filling based on what you like or what your refrigerator happens to be sheltering. Here are a few ideas to get the wheels turning:

★ Sautéed chorizo, onions, and poblano peppers

★ Leftover chicken or steak; pesto; and ricotta cheese

★ Mushrooms, spinach, sundried tomatoes, and feta

SKILLET SECRET

While it may make cleanup a snap, that nonstick pan could have harmful health effects. The chemicals that make the surface stickfree have been linked to infertility, thyroid disease, and high cholesterol. Stay safe by not overheating an empty nonstick pan or opt for a ceramic alternative. We like Green Pans (green-pan.com).

Smoked Salmon Sandwich

8 MINUTE MEAL! This breakfast sandwich is based on the famous everything bagels with lox of the New York Jewish deli canon; only this sandwich trades the bloated, carb-heavy bagel for fiber-rich whole-wheat bread.

- ¼ cup whipped cream cheese*
- 8 slices whole-wheat or 9-grain bread, toasted
- 2 Tbsp capers, rinsed and chopped
- ½ red onion, thinly sliced
- 2 cups mixed baby greens
- 1 large tomato, sliced
  Salt and black pepper to taste
- 8 oz smoked salmon

Spread 1 tablespoon of the cream cheese on each of four slices of toast. Top each with capers, onion, greens, and a slice or two of tomato. Lightly salt the tomato, then add as much pepper as you'd like (this sandwich cries out for a lot of it). Finish by draping a few slices of smoked salmon over the tomatoes and topping with the remaining slices of toasted bread.

5 POWER FOODS

4 SERVINGS

373 CALORIES

10 G FAT

3 G SAT. FAT

477 MG SODIUM

5 G FIBER

*Not only is whipped cream cheese easier to spread, it's also less calorie dense than the stuff that comes in a block.

Blueberry Pancakes

8 MINUTE MEAL! Using yogurt and cottage cheese to make these pancakes does two things: It brings extra protein to the breakfast table, and it helps produce the lightest, moistest pancakes you've ever tasted. And once you try this simple blueberry compote, you'll never go back to lackluster syrup again.

4 POWER FOODS

4 SERVINGS

315 CALORIES

6 G FAT

2 G SAT. FAT

497 MG SODIUM

7 G FIBER

*These can be just as easily made with white flour; you'll just sacrifice a few grams of fiber.

- 2 cups frozen wild blueberries
- ½ cup water
- ¼ cup sugar
- 1 cup plain Greek-style yogurt (such as Fage 2%)
- 1 cup low-fat cottage cheese or ricotta
- 3 eggs
  Juice of 1 lemon
- 1 cup white whole-wheat flour (we like King Arthur's)*
- ½ tsp baking soda
  Pinch of salt

Mix the blueberries, water, and sugar in a saucepan. Cook over low heat, stirring often, for 10 minutes or until the blueberries begin to break apart.

Whisk together the yogurt, cottage cheese, eggs, and lemon juice in a bowl. Mix the flour, baking soda, and salt in another bowl. Add the flour to the yogurt mixture and stir just until blended.

Heat a large skillet or sauté pan over medium-low heat. Coat with nonstick cooking spray and add the batter in large spoonfuls (about ¼ cup each). Flip the pancakes when the tops begin to bubble, 3 to 5 minutes, and cook the second side until browned. Serve with the warm blueberries.

NUTRITIONAL UPGRADE

Most supermarket syrups are junk, made almost entirely from high-fructose corn syrup and chemical additives designed to approximate a maple flavor. But real maple syrup can be prohibitively expensive. Solution? Fruit compote. Take a bag of frozen fruit (blueberries, strawberries, or mixed berries), dump into a saucepan with ½ cup water and ¼ cup sugar, and simmer for 10 minutes, until the fruit is warm and the mixture has thickened.

Lunch

The midday meal is the one most of us toss off—it's whatever's in the fridge, or whatever we can scrounge up at the local deli or fast food joint. But lunch is your best opportunity to really pack plenty of nutrition into your day. And for many 8-Hour dieters, it will be the breakfast meal. Make the most of it. Skip the salad bar, save your money, and try these instead.

Spinach and Ham Quiche

8 MINUTE MEAL!   Quiche is the ultimate culinary chameleon, not just because you can tweak different flavor combinations endlessly, but because it's as good for breakfast as it is for dinner. Let's split the difference and call it a stellar workday lunch, especially if flanked by a light side salad.

3 POWER FOODS

6 SERVINGS

282 CALORIES

18 G FAT

7 G SAT. FAT

467 MG SODIUM

1 G FIBER

1   frozen pie shell
1   Tbsp olive oil
1   clove garlic, minced
½   bunch spinach
2   oz smoked ham, cut into ¼-inch cubes
½   cup grated Swiss cheese, such as Gruyère
4   large eggs
¾   cup 1% milk
¼   cup half and half
½   tsp salt
      Pinch of nutmeg

Preheat oven to 375°F. When hot, place the pie shell on the middle rack and cook until lightly toasted, but not brown, about 8 minutes.

While the oven heats and the shell cooks, heat the olive oil in a large skillet or pot over medium heat. Add the garlic, cook for 30 seconds, then add the spinach. Cook until the spinach is fully wilted. In a large mixing bowl, combine with the ham, cheese, eggs, milk, half and half, and spinach, squeezing the spinach thoroughly beforehand to purge any excess water. Season with salt and a pinch of nutmeg.

Pour the egg mixture into the warm pastry shell. Bake in the oven until the quiche has browned lightly on top and a toothpick inserted into the center comes out clean, about 12 minutes.

Chinese Chicken Salad

This is fusion cuisine at its finest: a salad made with Asian ingredients popularized by an Austrian chef (Wolfgang Puck) cooking in a California restaurant (Spago in Beverly Hills). Thankfully its nutrient profile is as diverse as its roots, making for one powerful way to stave off midday hunger.

5 POWER FOODS

4 SERVINGS

242 CALORIES

6 G FAT

1 G SAT. FAT

387 MG SODIUM

5 G FIBER

- 1 head napa cabbage
- ½ head red cabbage
- ½ Tbsp sugar
- 2 cups chopped or shredded cooked chicken (freshly roasted or from a store-bought rotisserie chicken)
- ⅓ cup store-bought Asian-style vinaigrette (we like Annie's Organic Asian Sesame Vinaigrette)
- 1 cup fresh cilantro leaves
- 1 cup canned mandarin oranges, drained
- ¼ cup sliced almonds, toasted
  Salt and black pepper to taste

Slice the cabbages in half lengthwise and remove the cores. Slice them into thin strips. Toss with the sugar in a large bowl.

If the chicken is cold, toss with a few tablespoons of vinaigrette and heat in a microwave at 50 percent power. Add to the cabbage, along with the cilantro, oranges, almonds, and the remaining vinaigrette. Toss to combine. Season with salt and pepper.

Rotisserie Turkey with Cranberries, Avocado, and Goat Cheese

8 MINUTE MEAL! As good as this combination is in salad form, you could just as easily combine these ingredients on toasted whole-grain bread or stuff them inside a pita for a killer handheld lunch.

5 POWER FOODS

4 SERVINGS

324 CALORIES

17 G FAT

4 G SAT. FAT

306 MG SODIUM

4 G FIBER

- 12 oz sliced roast turkey
- 12 cups arugula (1 prewashed bag)
- ¼ cup dried cranberries
- 1 avocado, pitted, peeled, and sliced
- ¼ cup crumbled goat cheese
- ¼ cup walnuts, roughly chopped
- ¼ cup favorite vinaigrette (we like Marie's Balsamic Vinaigrette)
    Salt and black pepper to taste

Combine the turkey, arugula, cranberries, avocado, goat cheese, walnuts, vinaigrette, salt, and pepper in a large bowl, using your hands or two forks to fully incorporate the dressing.

Avocado-Tuna Salad

8 MINUTE MEAL! This dish uses ripe avocados as an edible salad bowl. The creaminess of the avocado means you don't need to drown your tuna in mayonnaise to make it tasty. For that matter, you don't even need to use tuna: leftover chicken, hard-boiled eggs, or lump crab meat would all work beautifully here.

4 POWER FOODS

4 SERVINGS

340 CALORIES

24 G FAT

4 G SAT. FAT

556 MG SODIUM

10 G FIBER

- 2 cans (5 oz each) tuna, drained
- ½ cup diced, seeded, and peeled cucumber
- ¼ cup minced red onion
- ¼ cup chopped cilantro
- 1 jalapeño pepper, minced
- 1 Tbsp soy sauce
- 1 Tbsp light mayonnaise
- 1 Tbsp sugar
- 1 tsp toasted sesame seeds (optional)
  Juice of 1 lime
  Salt
- 4 small ripe Hass avocados, halved and pitted

Combine the tuna, cucumber, onion, cilantro, jalapeño, soy sauce, mayonnaise, sugar, sesame seeds, and lime juice in a mixing bowl. Stir gently to combine. Lightly salt the flesh of the avocados, then divide the tuna mixture among the eight halves, spooning it directly into the bowls created by removing the pits.

Greek Salad

8 MINUTE MEAL!

The Greeks, true masters of the Mediterranean diet, know a thing or two about creating meals that are both intensely flavorful and insanely nutritious. Exhibit A below. This salad would be just as good made with canned tuna, chopped hard-boiled egg, or no main protein at all.

5 POWER FOODS

4 SERVINGS

355 CALORIES

22 G FAT

7 G SAT. FAT

570 MG SODIUM

5 G FIBER

2   cups shredded or chopped cooked chicken
1   large cucumber, peeled, seeded, and chopped
1   red bell pepper, chopped
4   Roma tomatoes, chopped
1   red onion, chopped
½   (14 to 16 oz) can garbanzo beans, drained
¾   cup crumbled feta
2   Tbsp red wine vinegar
1   tsp dried oregano
     Salt and black pepper to taste
¼   cup olive oil

Combine the chicken, cucumber, bell pepper, tomato, onion, beans, and feta in a large salad bowl. In a separate bowl, combine the vinegar and oregano with a few generous pinches of salt and pepper. Slowly drizzle in the olive oil, whisking to combine. Toss the dressing with the salad. You can serve now, but it's best to let this one sit in the fridge for 30 minutes or so, which gives all the ingredients a chance to get friendly.

Poor Man's Lobster Roll

8 MINUTE MEAL!

An ode to the great lobster rolls of the Maine coastline, which are as simple to make as they are satisfying to devour. This version, though, substitutes shrimp for lobster, cutting the price dramatically but maintaining the same sweet, ocean flavor.

3 POWER FOODS

4 SERVINGS

289 CALORIES

9 G FAT

1.5 G SAT. FAT

631 MG SODIUM

4 G FIBER

- 1 lb cooked shrimp
- 2 stalks celery, diced
- ½ small red onion, minced
- 2 Tbsp minced chives
- 2 Tbsp mayonnaise
  Juice of 1 lemon
- 1 tsp hot sauce (we like sriracha)
  Salt to taste
- 4 whole-wheat hot dog buns
  Chopped chives (optional)

Mix the shrimp, celery, onion, chives, mayo, lemon juice, hot sauce, and salt together in a bowl, stirring to incorporate carefully.

Heat a cast-iron skillet or sauté pan over medium heat. Add the hot dog buns and toast until the sides are nicely browned.

Divide the shrimp mixture among the rolls. Garnish with chopped chives, if desired.

Chicken Salad Sandwich with Curry and Raisins

Chicken salad routinely ranks as one of the worst sandwiches you can order at a deli because it is nothing but an excuse to lay on the mayo. This version cuts back on the gloppy stuff, but ratchets up flavor with sweet raisins, crunchy celery and vegetables, and a bit of curry to add an exotic touch and a boatload of antioxidants.

6 POWER FOODS

4 SERVINGS

414 CALORIES

11 G FAT

2 G SAT. FAT

688 MG SODIUM

7 G FIBER

- 3   Tbsp golden raisins
- 3   cups chopped cooked chicken
- 2   stalks celery, thinly sliced
- ½   onion, diced
- 1   carrot, shredded
- ½   tsp curry powder
- ¼   cup olive-oil mayonnaise
     Salt and black pepper to taste
- 4   large lettuce leaves (romaine, iceberg, or anything else)
- 8   slices whole-grain bread or English muffin halves, toasted
- 2   medium tomatoes, sliced

Cover the raisins with hot water and soak for at least 10 minutes (the warm water will help the raisins plump up); drain and place in a large bowl. Add the chicken, celery, onion, carrot, curry powder, and mayonnaise. Mix well and season with salt and pepper.

Place the lettuce leaves on top of four bread slices, then top with tomatoes, chicken salad, and the remaining bread.

Roast Beef and Cheddar with Horseradish Mayo

8 MINUTE MEAL!

When it comes to making great sandwiches, it's the little things that matter most. Here, that little thing is a simple horseradish sauce, the kind you might serve over a roast at the dinner table. Combined with sharp Cheddar and peppery arugula, it's enough to turn a standard weekday sandwich into something heroic.

5 POWER FOODS

4 SERVINGS

419 CALORIES

19 G FAT

8 G SAT. FAT

988 MG SODIUM

7 G FIBER

- 2 Tbsp olive-oil mayonnaise
- 2 Tbsp plain Greek-style yogurt (such as Fage 2%)
- 2 Tbsp prepared horseradish
- 1 clove garlic
- 1 Tbsp Dijon mustard
- 2 cups arugula
- 8 slices multigrain bread, lightly toasted
  Salt to taste
- 1 large tomato, sliced
- ½ red onion, very thinly sliced
- 1 lb deli roast beef
- 4 slices sharp Cheddar cheese

Combine the mayonnaise, yogurt, horseradish, garlic, and mustard in a mixing bowl.

Divide the arugula among four pieces of bread. Top with tomato (seasoned with a pinch of salt), sliced onion, roast beef, and cheese. Spread the top pieces of bread with a thick layer of the sauce to complete the sandwich.

Turkey, Bacon, Guacamole Sandwich

As great as guacamole is with chips, it's even better slathered on a sandwich. Swapping in the avocado all-star for mayo not only shaves 70 to 100 calories from your sandwich but also replaces low-quality fats with healthy monounsaturated ones. Turn guacamole into your spread of choice for turkey, chicken, and grilled steak sandwiches.

5 POWER FOODS

4 SERVINGS

471 CALORIES

18 G FAT

7 G SAT. FAT

1,685 MG SODIUM

4 G FIBER

*Fresh jalapeños will work, too. Be aware that they're spicier when fresh, so slice them thinly.

1	baguette or 4 individual sandwich rolls (preferably whole grain)
12	oz sliced turkey
4	slices Swiss cheese
1	large tomato, sliced
½	red onion, thinly sliced Pickled jalapeños, sliced*
4	strips bacon, cooked until crisp and patted dry
¼	cup Ultimate Guacamole (page 184) or store-bought guacamole, such as Wholly Guacamole

Preheat the broiler. Carefully slice the baguette in half horizontally and place on a large baking sheet. Layer the turkey and cheese on the bottom half of the bread.

Place the sheet in the oven 6" below the broiler. Broil for 2 to 3 minutes, until the cheese has just melted and both halves of the bread are hot, but not too brown and crunchy.

Remove from the oven and then layer the tomato, onion, jalapeños, and bacon on top of the turkey. Spread the top half of the baguette with the guacamole. Slice the baguette into 4 individual sandwiches and serve.

WEIGHT-LOSS WEAPON

Wholly Guacamole

Sure, this sandwich is best with homemade guacamole, but in case time is short or the avocados aren't ripe, this store-bought brand is a perfectly unadulterated rendition of a classic guac. Many "guacamole dips" are made, astoundingly, with less than 2 percent avocado and with a chemist's kit of food additives filling out much of the tub. But Wholly Guacamole uses just seven ingredients, the first being avocado—exactly as it should be. It contains just 25 calories per tablespoon; compare that with 90 calories for relatively flavorless mayonnaise, and you start to realize why we love this product so much.

Pesto Tuna Melt

8 MINUTE MEAL!

Ahh, the tuna melt: Has any sandwich squandered more potential more consistently than this fishy fiasco? The recipe used by most establishments tells all: 2 parts mayo to 1 part tuna. This recipe replaces the bulk of the mayo with a considerably healthier supporting cast: pesto, lemon juice, olives, and onions. That means you can taste something other than fat when you're eating it and feel something other than fat when you're through.

4 POWER FOODS

4 SERVINGS

411 CALORIES

16 G FAT

3 G SAT. FAT

804 MG SODIUM

15 G FIBER

*When it comes to whole-wheat bread, nothing beats Martin's Whole Wheat Potato Bread.

2 cans (5 oz each) tuna, drained
1 small red onion, diced
¼ cup chopped green olives
2 Tbsp olive-oil mayonnaise
2 Tbsp bottled pesto
1 Tbsp capers, rinsed and chopped
   Juice of 1 lemon
8 slices whole-wheat bread*
2 oz fresh mozzarella, sliced (you can use low-fat shredded mozzarella, too)
1 large tomato, sliced
   About 1 tsp olive oil

In a mixing bowl, combine the tuna, onion, olives, mayo, pesto, capers, and lemon juice and stir to combine. Layer the bottom half of four slices of bread with mozzarella, then top with the tuna mixture, tomato slices, and remaining slices of bread.

Preheat a cast-iron or nonstick pan over medium heat. Coat with a thin layer of olive oil and cook the sandwiches for 2 to 3 minutes per side, until the bread is toasted and the cheese is melted.

Chicken and White Bean Chili

Few foods travel better than chili. That means you can make up a big batch over the weekend (try it in the slow cooker if you want to make your life even easier) and have a hearty, protein- and fiber-filled lunch at your disposal all week long.

4 POWER FOODS

8 SERVINGS

459 CALORIES

19 G FAT

5 G SAT. FAT

700 MG SODIUM

5 G FIBER

*The mix of ground and chopped chicken gives this chili a more interesting texture, but if you prefer one over the other, simply use 2 pounds of your chicken of choice.

- 1 Tbsp olive oil
- 2 yellow onions, chopped
- 4 cloves garlic, minced
- 1 lb boneless, skinless chicken thighs, cut into small pieces*
- 1 lb lean ground chicken
- 1 can (7 oz) roasted green chiles
- 1 tsp ground cumin
- 1 tsp dried oregano
- ¼ tsp cayenne pepper
- 4 cups low-sodium chicken stock
- 1 can (14 to 16 oz each) white kidney beans (also called cannellini and great northern beans), drained
  Salt and black pepper to taste
  Fresh cilantro, shredded cheese, diced onion, sour cream, and/or sliced jalapeños, for serving

Heat the oil in a large pot over medium heat. Add the onion and garlic and cook for about 3 minutes, until the onion is translucent. Add the chicken thighs, ground chicken, chiles, cumin, oregano, and cayenne. Sauté until the chicken is mostly cooked through, about 8 minutes. Add the stock and beans. Turn the heat down to low.

Simmer uncovered for at least 20 minutes, or longer if you have the patience. Taste the chili and adjust the seasoning with salt and pepper. Serve with any combination of the garnishes.

Sesame Noodles with Chicken and Peanuts

8 MINUTE MEAL!

This nutrient-dense Asian-style noodle dish is like revenge: It's best served cold. Make it in the morning and stash it in the fridge until you're ready to feast.

5 POWER FOODS

4 SERVINGS

348 CALORIES

9 G FAT

2 G SAT. FAT

361 MG SODIUM

4 G FIBER

6	oz whole-wheat fettuccine
2	tsp toasted sesame oil, plus more for noodles
	Dash of rice wine vinegar
	Juice of 1 lime
2	Tbsp warm water
1½	Tbsp chunky peanut butter
1½	Tbsp low-sodium soy sauce
2	tsp chili sauce, such as sriracha
2	cups shredded chicken breast
1	red or yellow bell pepper, sliced
2	cups sugar snap peas
1	cup cooked and shelled edamame (optional)
	Chopped peanuts, sesame seeds, or chopped scallions (optional)

Bring a large pot of salted water to a boil and cook the pasta according to package instructions. Drain the pasta and toss in a large bowl with a bit of sesame oil and rice wine vinegar to keep the noodles from sticking.

Combine the lime juice, water, peanut butter, soy sauce, chili sauce, and sesame oil in a microwave-safe mixing bowl. Microwave for 45 seconds, then stir to create a uniform sauce.

Add the sauce to the noodles and toss to mix. Stir in the chicken, bell pepper, sugar snaps, and edamame if using. Top individual servings with peanuts, sesame seeds, or scallions, if you like.

Southwestern Turkey Burger

8 MINUTE MEAL!

Whereas beef burgers are best left relatively un-adorned, turkey burgers demand a more aggressive culinary strategy. Thus you'll roll this burger in blackening seasoning, slick it with a spicy-cool chipotle mayonnaise, and top it with avocado and fresh salsa.

5 POWER FOODS

4 SERVINGS

446 CALORIES

19 G FAT

6 G SAT. FAT

1,235 MG SODIUM

6 G FIBER

2   Tbsp olive-oil mayonnaise
1   Tbsp chipotle pepper*
1   Tbsp lime juice
1   lb ground turkey
1   Tbsp bottled blackening seasoning
4   slices pepper or regular Monterey jack cheese
    Salt and black pepper to taste
1   avocado, peeled, pitted, and thinly sliced
1   cup favorite salsa
4   English muffins (preferable whole grain) or potato rolls, lightly toasted

*Chipotle peppers are smoked jalape-ños that come sold in cans of spicy-sweet adobo sauce. In a pinch, substitute your favorite hot sauce.

In a mixing bowl, combine the mayo, chipotle, and lime juice. Reserve.

Preheat a grill, grill pan, or cast-iron skillet over medium heat. Gently form the turkey into four equal patties (being careful not to overwork the meat, which makes for dense, tough burgers). Season both sides of the burger with blackening seasoning, plus salt and black pepper.

Cook the burger until a nice dark crust has formed on the bottom side, about 4 minutes. Flip and immediately cover with the cheese. Continue cooking until the cheese is melted and the burger is just firm to the touch, about 4 minutes more. Top four English muffin halves with avocado slices and salsa, then place a burger on top of each. Spoon the sauce over the burgers and serve.

WEIGHT-LOSS WEAPON
Caramelized Onions

Caramelized onions, juicy and sweet and flavorful, make for a potent low-calorie replacement to fatty condiments on burgers and sandwiches. Thinly slice two large yellow or red onions. Heat a tablespoon of oil in a large saucepan or pot over low heat and add the onions, plus a pinch of salt. Cook with the lid on, stirring occasionally for 20 minutes, until very soft and lightly browned. Add a tablespoon of balsamic vinegar in the last few minutes to intensify the sweetness, if you like. These onions will keep covered in the refrigerator for up to a week.

The Ultimate Burger

8 MINUTE MEAL! A great burger doesn't need crazy condiments or other high-calorie bells and whistles. It just needs excellent, fresh-ground beef cooked to perfection. Use this recipe as your base for all other burgers you cook.

10 oz ground sirloin
10 oz ground brisket
1 tsp salt
1 tsp freshly cracked pepper
4 hamburger buns (preferably Martin's Potato Rolls*), toasted
2 cups arugula
½ cup caramelized onions (see the opposite page)

3 POWER FOODS

4 SERVINGS

358 CALORIES
10 G FAT
3 G SAT. FAT
831 MG SODIUM
4 G FIBER

*Martin's Potato Rolls aren't just the perfect size (not too big or bready) for the burger—they also pack 3 grams of fiber apiece.

Heat a grill or stovetop grill pan until hot. Combine the sirloin, brisket, salt, and pepper in a bowl and gently mix. Form into four patties. Caution: Overworking the meat or packing your patties too tightly can make tough burgers.

Cook the burgers for 2 to 3 minutes and flip. Cook on the other side for another 2 to 3 minutes, until nicely charred on the outside but still medium-rare to medium within. (The center of the patty should be firm but easily yielding—like a Nerf football.)

After you remove the burgers, toast the buns briefly. Divide the arugula among the buns and top with the burgers and onions.

Dinner

The perfect dinner is something that takes little time to whip up—hey, it's a long commute home each day!—but that gives you the feeling that you're wrapping your day up in style. For the 8-Hour Diet, the perfect dinner is also one that's plenty filling, to see you through your next stretch between meals.

Grilled Fish Tacos with Mango Salsa

Fish tacos are traditionally battered and fried, but the spicy crust of blackened mahimahi paired against the creamy cool of an avocado-mango salsa is a strong reminder of just how boring fried food can be. If there is a recipe that packs more flavor into fewer calories, we haven't seen it.

1	mango, peeled, pitted, and cubed*
1	avocado, pitted, peeled, and cubed
½	red onion, finely chopped
	Juice of 1 lime, plus wedges for garnish
	Chopped fresh cilantro
	Salt and black pepper to taste
	Canola oil
2	large mahimahi fillets (1½ lbs total)
1	Tbsp blackening spice
8	corn tortillas
2	cups finely shredded red cabbage

5 POWER FOODS

4 SERVINGS

405 CALORIES

11 G FAT

2 G SAT. FAT

615 MG SODIUM

8 G FIBER

*No ripe mangoes at the super-market? Both pineapple and peaches would make perfect substitutes.

Mix the mango, avocado, onion, and the lime juice in a bowl. Season with cilantro, salt, and pepper.

Heat a grill or stovetop grill pan until hot. Drizzle a light coating of oil over the fish and rub on the blackening spice. Cook the fish, undisturbed, for 4 minutes. Carefully flip with a spatula and cook for another 4 minutes. Remove.

Warm the tortillas on the grill for 1 to 2 minutes or wrap in damp paper towels and microwave for 1 minute until warm and pliable.

Break the fish into chunks and divide among the warm tortillas. Top with the cabbage and the mango salsa. Serve with the lime wedges.

Loaded Alfredo with Chicken and Vegetables

In the century or so since Alfredo started dressing his noodles, his dish has taken on a thick coating of heavy cream and about 800 extra calories. This version, made with béchamel and loaded with lean protein and vegetables, takes the flab out of Alfredo.

5 POWER FOODS

4 SERVINGS

612 CALORIES

15 G FAT

7 G SAT. FAT

297 MG SODIUM

12 G FIBER

- 2 Tbsp unsalted butter
- 3 Tbsp flour
- 3 cups 2% milk
- 2 cloves garlic, chopped
- 2 Tbsp grated Parmesan
  Salt and black pepper to taste
- ½ Tbsp olive oil
- 2 cups bite-size broccoli florets
- 8 oz cremini mushrooms, sliced
- ¼ cup chopped sundried tomatoes
- 8 oz cooked chicken breast, thinly sliced (store-bought rotisserie chicken works well)
- 12 oz whole-wheat fettuccine (we like Ronzoni Healthy Harvest)

To make the white sauce, melt the butter in a saucepan over medium-low heat. Whisk in the flour. Cook for 1 minute. Slowly whisk in the milk to prevent any lumps from forming. Add the garlic and simmer, whisking often, for 10 to 15 minutes, or until nicely thickened. Stir in the Parmesan and season with salt and pepper. Keep warm.

Heat the oil in a large skillet or sauté pan over medium-high heat. Add the broccoli and cook for 3 to 4 minutes. Add the mushrooms and tomatoes. Cook for 5 minutes, or until the vegetables have lightly caramelized. Stir in the chicken. Season with salt and pepper.

Meanwhile, cook the pasta according to the package instructions. Drain, reserving 1 cup of the cooking water. Return the pasta to the pot, add the sauce and the chicken mixture, and toss to coat. If the sauce is too thick, add some of the pasta water to thin it. Serve immediately.

Honey-Mustard Salmon with Roasted Asparagus

A piece of spanking fresh salmon needs little adornment, but this quick honey mustard is so perfectly suited to the rich flavor of the salmon that it's likely to become your fall-back method for doing fish at home. This is a recipe kids—even the picky, nonfish-eating ones—will love.

3 POWER FOODS

4 SERVINGS

450 CALORIES

28 G FAT

7 G SAT. FAT

530 MG SODIUM

2 G FIBER

- 1 bunch asparagus
- ½ Tbsp olive oil
  Salt and black pepper to taste
- 1 Tbsp butter
- 1 Tbsp brown sugar
- 2 Tbsp Dijon mustard
- 1 Tbsp honey
- 1 Tbsp soy sauce
- 4 salmon fillets (6 oz each)
- 1 tsp toasted sesame seeds (optional)

Preheat the oven to 450°F. Toss the asparagus with the olive oil, plus salt and black pepper to taste. Lay the spears out on a baking sheet and reserve.

Combine the butter and brown sugar in a bowl and microwave for 30 seconds, until the butter and sugar have melted together. Stir in the mustard, honey, and soy sauce. Season the salmon with salt and pepper and rub all over with half of the honey-mustard mixture. Position the salmon on top of the asparagus on the baking sheet and place in the middle of the oven.

Roast the salmon until the fish flakes with gentle pressure from your finger (but before the white fat begins to form on the surface), about 8 to 10 minutes. Remove, brush the salmon with more of the honey mustard, and serve with the asparagus. Top with sesame seeds, if using.

Cornmeal Catfish with Corn Salsa

8 MINUTE MEAL! This Southwestern-style treat can be cooked up in a matter of minutes on a busy weeknight. Toast the corn, combine with the avocado and black beans, and sear the fish on the stovetop. The combination of protein, healthy fat, and fiber is the perfect way to get you through the 12 hours until your next meal.

4 POWER FOODS

4 SERVINGS

530 CALORIES

25 G FAT

4 G SAT. FAT

408 MG SODIUM

9 G FIBER

- 4 tsp canola oil
- 1 ear corn, kernels removed from the cob
- 1 can (16 oz) black beans, rinsed and drained
- 1 avocado, pitted, and cut into cubes
  Juice of 1 lime, plus wedges for garnish
- 1 jalapeño, minced
  Salt and black pepper
- 1 cup cornmeal
- ⅛ tsp cayenne pepper
- 4 catfish or tilapia fillets (6 oz each)

Heat 1 teaspoon of the oil in a medium saucepan over medium-high heat. Add the corn kernels and cook, stirring occasionally, until they're lightly browned, about 3 minutes. Add the beans and warm through. Transfer to a bowl and stir in the avocado, lime juice, and jalapeño; season with salt and pepper.

Pour the cornmeal onto a large plate; season with the cayenne, 1 teaspoon salt, and ¼ teaspoon pepper. Dredge the fillets in the cornmeal until evenly coated.

Heat the remaining 3 teaspoons of oil in a large nonstick skillet or sauté pan over medium heat. When the oil is hot, add the catfish and cook for 4 to 5 minutes per side, until the coating is golden and crispy and the fish flakes easily. Serve the fish topped with the salsa, along with additional lime wedges, if you like.

Halibut in a Bag

The French call it *en papillote;* the Italians, *in cartoccio.* Forget about the fancy monikers—just know that cooking in a bag is a technique that combines health, flavor, and convenience as effectively as any cooking method in the kitchen. By adding a bit of liquid (wine, broth, lemon juice), you create a perfect steaming environment for chicken, fish, and seafood. Toss in tomatoes, onions, zucchini—anything that will cook in 15 minutes or less—to bolster the flavor. The best part? No cleanup.

4 POWER FOODS

2 SERVINGS

361 CALORIES

12 G FAT

2 G SAT. FAT

1,119 MG SODIUM

7 G FIBER

*Fennel is a bulbous vegetable with a cool anise undertone. If you're not a fan of licorice (or don't want to spend $3 on a fennel bulb for this recipe), yellow onion can stand in.

- 2   fillets of halibut or other firm white fish (5 oz each)
- 1   jar (8 oz) marinated artichoke hearts, drained
- 1   cup cherry tomatoes
- 2   Tbsp chopped kalamata olives
- ½   medium fennel bulb, thinly sliced*
- 1   lemon, half cut into thin slices, the other half cut into quarters
- ½   Tbsp olive oil
- ¼   cup dry white wine
     Salt and black pepper to taste

Preheat the oven to 400°F.

Take 2 large sheets of parchment paper or foil, place a fillet in the center of each, and top equally with the artichokes, tomatoes, olives, fennel, and lemon slices. Drizzle with the olive oil and wine; season with salt and pepper. Fold the paper or foil over the fish and seal by tightly rolling up the edges, creating a secure pouch. It's important the packets are fully sealed, so that the steam created inside can't escape.

Place the pouches on a baking sheet in the center of the oven and bake for 20 to 25 minutes, depending on how thick the fish is. Serve with the remaining lemon wedges.

Grilled Pork and Peaches

8 MINUTE MEAL!

Pork and fruit have been dance partners since the dawn of time: pork and prunes, chops and applesauce, prosciutto and melon. This is the latest iteration of this long-time collaboration—a thick chop grilled until juicy, then topped with a salsa of grilled peaches, red onions, and blue cheese.

5 POWER FOODS

4 SERVINGS

496 CALORIES

29 G FAT

9 G SAT. FAT

552 MG SODIUM

3 G FIBER

- 4   thick-cut (1"), bone-in pork chops (8 oz each)*
       Olive oil
       Salt and black pepper to taste
- 2   firm peaches or nectarines, halved and pitted
- 2   Tbsp pine nuts, toasted
- 1   small red onion, thinly sliced
- ½   cup crumbled blue cheese
- 1   Tbsp balsamic vinegar

*Prepackaged pork chops are cut too thin, so they dry out easily. Have the butcher cut them thick and on the bone, which imparts moisture and flavor during cooking.

Heat a grill to hot. Brush the pork with olive oil and season with salt and pepper. Grill for 4 to 5 minutes on each side. The outside should be charred (not burned), but the meat should be light pink in the middle.

While the chops cook, brush the peach halves with oil and add them to the grill, cut side down. Grill for 5 minutes or until soft. Remove, slice, and toss with the pine nuts, onion, blue cheese, and vinegar; season with salt and pepper. Top each chop with half of the peach mixture and serve.

Seared Sirloin with Red Wine Mushrooms

Most people cook their steaks outdoors, but a cast-iron skillet set on the stovetop allows you to cook the steak more quickly and with more accuracy. And it provides the foundation to build a quick pan sauce to pour over the beef. This move will make you feel like a professional chef without having the prodigious belly of one.

2 POWER FOODS

4 SERVINGS

329 CALORIES

10 G FAT

3 G SAT. FAT

366 MG SODIUM

1 G FIBER

1	Tbsp olive oil
4	sirloin steaks or petite filets (6 oz each)
	Salt and black pepper to taste
2	shallots, minced
2	cloves garlic, minced
½	lb white or cremini mushrooms, cleaned, stems removed, and sliced
1	cup red wine
1	cup low-sodium beef stock
2	tsp fresh rosemary, chopped

Preheat the oven to 400°F. Heat the oil in a large cast-iron or oven-safe skillet over high heat. Season the steaks with salt and plenty of black pepper and add to the hot pan. Sear the first side for 3 to 4 minutes, until a deep brown crust has developed, then flip. Place the pan in the oven to finish cooking (about 6 to 8 minutes for medium rare; an instant-read thermometer inserted into the thickest part will read 135°F). Remove from the oven and transfer the steaks to a cutting board to rest.

Using a potholder, place the pan back on the stove over medium heat. Add the shallots, garlic, and mushrooms and cook for 3 to 4 minutes, until the mushrooms have begun to caramelize. Add the red wine and the stock, using a wooden spoon to scrape the bottom of the pan. Cook for another 2 to 3 minutes, until the alcohol has burned off and the liquid has reduced by about half. Stir in the rosemary.

Divide the steaks among four plates, top with mush-rooms, and spoon on the sauce. Serve with a side of Parmesan-Roasted Broccoli (page 182) to boost fiber.

Hoisin Beef Kebab

8 MINUTE MEAL!

Meat, stick, fire: Few dishes are as primal and satisfying as a flame-licked skewer loaded to the hilt with fresh ingredients. The key to this one is the hoisin, an Asian ketchup-like condiment perfect for sauces and stir-fries.

3 POWER FOODS

4 SERVINGS

231 CALORIES

8 G FAT

2 G SAT. FAT

368 MG SODIUM

3 G FIBER

- 2 Tbsp hoisin sauce
- 1 Tbsp low-sodium soy sauce
- 2 tsp dark or toasted sesame oil
- 1 tsp chili sauce or paste, such as sriracha
- 1 lb sirloin, cut into ¾" pieces
- 8 scallion whites, chopped into ½" chunks
- 20 small mushroom caps
- 20 cherry tomatoes
- 8 wooden skewers, soaked in water for 20 minutes

Preheat a grill. Combine the hoisin, soy sauce, sesame oil, and chili sauce in a bowl and mix thoroughly. Transfer half to a separate bowl.

Thread the beef, scallion, mushrooms, and tomatoes in an alternating pattern onto the skewers. Use a brush to paint the skewers with some of the hoisin glaze. When the grill is hot, add the skewers and cook for 3 to 4 minutes per side, basting with a bit more of the sauce as you go. The skewers are done when the meat and vegetables are lightly charred and the beef is firm but still yielding to the touch.

Brush the kebabs with the reserved glaze before serving.

IMPROVISING SAUCES

Making a killer sauce on the fly for the grill is easier than most think. Start with a base with a well-rounded flavor: Ketchup, Dijon, hoisin all work. Then mix in other liquids or condiments that add strong single flavor notes: honey for sweetness, vinegar for acid, soy sauce for salt, sriracha for heat. Finally, turn to the spice cabinet to bring it all together. Chili powder, garlic and onion salts, cumin, brown sugar, mustard powder, and cayenne are all common elements of barbecue sauces and any could be the finishing touch for your next masterpiece.

Chicken Tacos with Salsa Verde

8 MINUTE MEAL! Supermarket rotisserie chickens are a gift to cooks with little time to spare. They can be devoured straight from the container, of course, but remove the skin and shred the meat and you have an amazing building block for salads, sandwiches, and insanely delicious 5-minute tacos.

8 corn tortillas
3 cups shredded rotisserie chicken (about three-fourths of a store-bought chicken)*
1½ cups bottled salsa verde
½ cup crumbled Cotija or feta cheese
1 medium red onion, minced
1 cup chopped fresh cilantro
2 limes, quartered

Heat the tortillas in a large skillet or sauté pan until lightly toasted. Combine the chicken with the salsa in a large mixing bowl, then divide evenly among the tortillas. Top with crumbled cheese, onion, and cilantro. Serve with lime wedges.

3 POWER FOODS
4 SERVINGS

389 CALORIES
13 G FAT
4.5 G SAT. FAT
800 MG SODIUM
5 G FIBER

*Be sure to remove the skin first. As delicious as it may be, its finer points will be lost in the salsa-strewn meat itself, so you may as well save the calories.

Chili-Mango Chicken

8 MINUTE MEAL! The wok is a powerful weapon of mass reduction, capable of producing lean, intensely flavorful dinners in a matter of minutes. Follow the basic technique below, but feel free to switch up the meat and vegetables to suit your tastes.

3 POWER FOODS

4 SERVINGS

242 CALORIES

8 G FAT

2 G SAT. FAT

265 MG SODIUM

2 G FIBER

- 1 lb boneless, skinless chicken thighs, chopped into ½" pieces
- 1 Tbsp cornstarch
- 1 Tbsp low-sodium soy sauce
- ½ Tbsp sesame oil
- ½ Tbsp peanut or canola oil
- 1 red onion, chopped
- 1 Tbsp grated or minced fresh ginger
- 2 cups sugar snap peas or green beans
- 1 mango, peeled, pitted, and chopped
- 1 Tbsp chili garlic sauce (preferably sambal oleek)
  Black pepper to taste

Combine the chicken, cornstarch, soy sauce, and sesame oil in a mixing bowl and let sit for 10 minutes.

Heat the peanut oil in a wok or large skillet over high heat. Add the onion and ginger and cook for 1 to 2 minutes, until the onion is translucent. Add the sugar snaps and stir-fry for 1 minute, using a metal spatula to keep the vegetables in near-constant motion. Add the chicken, along with its marinade, and stir-fry for about 2 minutes, until the meat begins to brown on the outside. Add the mango, chili sauce, and black pepper and stir-fry for 1 minute longer, until the chicken is cooked through and the mango has softened into a near sauce-like consistency. Serve over brown rice.

Asian Chicken Packet

Another example of how easy and awesome it is to cook your dinner inside a few sheets of aluminum foil. Feel free to change up the vegetables (broccoli, green beans, and button mushrooms work great) and the chicken (why not cod or snapper?) to fit your tastes; it's the technique, plus the powerful base of soy, mirin, and ginger, that makes this such a satisfying dinner.

3 POWER FOODS

4 SERVINGS

239 CALORIES

4.5 G FAT

1 G SAT. FAT

633 MG SODIUM

2 G FIBER

- 4 boneless, skinless chicken breasts (about 6 oz each)
- 12 spears asparagus, ends removed, chopped
- 4 oz shitake mushrooms, stems removed
- 1 Tbsp grated fresh ginger
- 2 Tbsp low-sodium soy sauce
- 2 Tbsp mirin (sweetened sake), sake, or sweet white wine
  Salt and black pepper to taste

Preheat the oven to 400°F.

Lay four large (18" × 12") pieces of aluminum foil on the kitchen counter and fold each into thirds. Place a chicken breast in the center third of each piece, then scatter the asparagus, mushrooms, and ginger over each. Drizzle with the soy sauce and mirin and season with a small pinch of salt (remember, soy sauce already packs plenty of sodium) and black pepper. Fold the outer two sections of the foil over the chicken, then roll up the ends toward the center to create a fully sealed packet.

Arrange the packets on a large baking sheet and bake for 15 minutes, depending on the thickness of the chicken breast. Place each packet directly on a plate and serve.

Curry with Cauliflower and Butternut Squash

You know you've got a great vegetarian dish when a hard-core carnivore wouldn't miss the meat. One bite of this complex curry—rich with coconut milk, garbanzo beans, and soft cubes of butternut squash—and it's safe to say that even the most dedicated meat eaters will be happy to take a night off.

4 POWER FOODS

4 SERVINGS

267 CALORIES

9 G FAT

5 G SAT. FAT

563 MG SODIUM

9 G FIBER

*Carrots or potatoes would both be perfect substitutes for the squash, just in case butternut is not in season.

½ Tbsp canola oil
1 medium red onion, diced
½ Tbsp minced fresh ginger
2 cups cubed butternut squash*
1 head cauliflower, cut into florets
1 can (14 to 16 oz) garbanzo beans (aka chickpeas), drained
1 jalapeño pepper, minced
1 Tbsp yellow curry powder
1 can (14 oz) diced tomatoes
1 can (14 oz) light coconut milk
   Juice of 1 lime
   Salt and black pepper to taste
   Chopped cilantro

Heat the oil in a large sauté pan or pot over medium heat. Add the onion and ginger and cook for about 2 minutes, until the onion is soft and translucent. Add the squash, cauliflower, garbanzos, jalapeño, and curry powder. Cook for 2 minutes, until the curry powder is fragrant and coats the vegetables evenly. Stir in the tomatoes and coconut milk and turn the heat down to low. Simmer for 15 to 20 minutes, until the vegetables are tender. Add the lime juice and season with salt and black pepper. Serve garnished with the chopped cilantro.

Shrimp Scampi

8 MINUTE MEAL! One of the fastest, leanest meals imaginable gets a bit healthier with the addition of lightly wilted spinach and a scattering of sundried tomatoes. Serve as is or over the top of a small portion of whole-wheat linguine or quinoa.

4 POWER FOODS

4 SERVINGS

170 CALORIES

5 G FAT

1 G SAT. FAT

403 MG SODIUM

2 G FIBER

1 Tbsp olive oil
3 cloves garlic, minced
  Pinch red pepper flakes
1 small red onion, thinly sliced
1 lb medium shrimp, peeled and deveined*
  Salt and black pepper to taste
4 cups baby spinach
¼ cup chopped sundried tomatoes (softened in hot water for 10 minutes before cooking)
  Zest and juice from 1 lemon

*Farmed shrimp from Thailand and other parts of Asia are often processed in squalid conditions. Whenever possible, look for wild-caught shrimp.

Heat the olive oil in a large skillet over medium-high heat. Add the garlic and pepper flakes and cook until the garlic is light brown, about 30 seconds. Add the onion and continue cooking until translucent.

CHANGE IT UP

Scampi need not be confined to shrimp cooked in garlic butter. Consider this version as a base, one that can benefit from a number of tweaks and additions. Here are a few variations to try.

★ ½ lb white or cremini mushrooms, sliced
★ Ground turkey sautéed with ginger, garlic, and soy sauce
★ 1 small jar marinated artichoke hearts
★ ½ cup roasted red pepper strips

Season the shrimp with a pinch of salt and add to the pan. Cook, stirring occasionally, until the shrimp are just pink. Stir in the spinach and sundried tomatoes and cook until the spinach is just wilted, about 30 seconds. Remove from the heat, stir in the lemon zest and lemon juice. Season with salt and pepper.

Super Supreme Pizza

Why wait for the delivery dude when you can have a cheaper, healthier, and more delicious pizza in half the time? This pizza has all the bells and whistles of a fully loaded pie, but because the crust is thin and the ingredients are carefully chosen, you end up with a pizza with a fraction of the calories.

6 POWER FOODS

4 SERVINGS

507 CALORIES

24 G FAT

8 G SAT. FAT

1,413 MG SODIUM

7 G FIBER

*Fresh basil is a perfect pizza garnish, but unless you have other uses for it, it's probably not worth the extra $2 or $3 price tag.

12"	Boboli whole-wheat thin pizza crust
1	cup tomato-basil pasta sauce (we like Muir Glen)
2	cups shredded part-skim mozzarella
15	slices turkey pepperoni
½	cup sliced onion
½	cup chopped roasted red peppers
½	cup chopped green olives
2	cloves garlic, minced
½	tsp red pepper flakes
1	jar (6 oz) artichoke hearts, drained
1	cup fresh basil leaves (optional)*

Preheat the oven to 400°F. Cover the crust with the sauce and then cheese. Sprinkle with the pepperoni, onion, peppers, olives, garlic, pepper flakes, and artichokes.

Bake for 12 to 15 minutes, until the cheese is melted and bubbling. Top with the basil (if using) and serve immediately.

WEIGHT-LOSS WEAPON
Boboli Whole-Wheat Crust

For years, Boboli has provided time-starved Americans with an alternative to delivery pizza. Problem is, most Americans opt for Boboli's regular crust, which is thick and doughy and thus overloaded with calories and carbs. Thankfully, they offer a whole-wheat, thin-crust alternative that not only reduces calories but also boosts fiber, maximizing the satiating effect of the pizza. If you'd rather make personal pizzas, try whole wheat English muffins or perfectly thin pita bread.

Grilled Steak Fajitas

On paper, fajitas sound like a brilliant way to avoid the more obvious pitfalls of a border crossing. Too bad most chains across the country—from Chili's to Applebee's to Baja Fresh—put out versions with more than 1,000 calories and a day's worth of sodium in every serving. These are the fajitas of your dreams: juicy grilled steak, charred peppers and onions, and plenty of fixings to stuff into your tortilla, but none of the four-digit danger of the average restaurant specimen.

6 POWER FOODS

4 SERVINGS

518 CALORIES

28 G FAT

8 G SAT. FAT

471 MG SODIUM

7 G FIBER

1   chipotle pepper in adobo
2   cloves garlic
1   tsp chili powder
¼   tsp cumin
    Juice of two limes
1   Tbsp sugar
¼   cup vegetable or canola oil
1   lb flank steak
    Salt and black pepper to taste
1   large sweet onion, sliced into ¼-inch rings
2   large bell peppers (a mix of green and red is best), pitted and quartered
    Ultimate Guacamole (see page 184) or use store-bought such as Wholly Guacamole
    Your favorite salsa (we like Muir Glen Cilantro Lime Salsa)
    Shredded Jack cheese
8   small corn tortillas, warm

Combine the chipotle, garlic, chili powder, cumin, lime juice, sugar, and oil in a food processor or blender. Puree until you have a smooth, uniform sauce. Combine with the steak in a sealable plastic bag and marinate in the refrigerator for at least 1 hour, and up to 4, before cooking.

Preheat a grill over high heat. Remove the steak from the marinade and pat dry with a paper towel. Season all over with salt and black pepper and grill for 4 to 5 minutes per side, until a crust has formed and the meat is firm but yielding to the touch. While the steak cooks, grill the onions and peppers until soft and caramelized.

After the steak has rested for at least 5 minutes, slice into thin pieces against the natural grain of the meat. Roughly chop the onions and peppers. Serve the steak and vegetables with guacamole, salsa, cheese, and warm tortillas.

Six Hunger-Squashing Snacks

The rule of snacks on the 8-Hour Diet is simple: Snack as much as you want, as long as you're within your 8-hour window. But you'll get the maximum weight loss and health benefits if you pack those snacks with nutrition. Here's how.

Parmesan-Roasted Broccoli

This simple roasting technique can be applied to any of a dozen different vegetables: asparagus, cauliflower, Brussels sprouts, red potatoes. Of course, the times will vary depending on the vegetable of choice (asparagus will be done in less than 10 minutes; potatoes will take closer to 30), but the results are uniformly satisfying. Any and all taste just as good at room temperature as they do fresh out of the oven, so bake up a batch and bring these with you on the go.

4 SERVINGS

100 CALORIES

5 G FAT

1.5 G SAT. FAT

272 MG SODIUM

4 G FIBER

1 head broccoli, cut into florets, bottom part of the stem removed
1 Tbsp olive oil
   Salt and black pepper to taste
¼ cup grated Parmesan cheese

Preheat oven to 450°F. Toss broccoli with olive oil, salt, and pepper and spread out evenly on a baking sheet. Roast in the oven until the broccoli is tender and lightly browned, about 12 minutes. Remove from the oven, toss with the cheese, and serve.

CHANGE IT UP

Hummus is dying to be embellished. The best part about making it from scratch at home (besides the money you'll save) is that you can punch it up however you like. Try these additions:

★ 5 or 6 whole roasted garlic cloves
★ ½ cup bottled roasted red peppers
★ ¼ cup chopped black olives
★ ¼ cup sundried tomatoes, minced

Hummus

Sure, you can find packaged hummus in nearly every market in America these days, but this version is gloriously simple and deeply delicious. Make a double batch and keep it in the fridge all week.

3 whole-wheat pitas, cut into wedges
1 can (14 to 16 oz) garbanzo beans (aka chickpeas), drained
2 Tbsp tahini*
  Juice of 1 lemon
2 cloves garlic, minced
½ tsp cumin
½ tsp salt
2 Tbsp olive oil

Preheat the oven to 400°F. Place the pita wedges on a baking sheet and bake for 10 minutes, until hot and lightly crisped.

Combine the beans, tahini, lemon juice, garlic, cumin, and salt in a food processor and puree. With the motor running, drizzle in the olive oil until the hummus has a thick, creamy consistency. If the mixture is still too thick, add a bit of water to thin it out. Serve with the toasted pita wedges. Keeps in the refrigerator for up to a week.

6 SERVINGS

315
CALORIES

13
G FAT

2
G SAT. FAT

633
MG SODIUM

7
G FIBER

*Tahini is a paste made from ground sesame seeds. It is easy to find these days, but if you can't, try 1 tablespoon of smooth peanut butter for the 2 tablespoons of tahini here.

Ultimate Guacamole

Companies like Wholly Guacamole make excellent, unadulterated versions of guacamole that are perfect in a pinch. But when it comes down to it, nothing is quite as good as homemade guac.

- ¼ cup chopped cilantro
- 2 cloves garlic, minced
  Salt to taste
- 2 ripe avocados, pitted and peeled*
- ¼ cup minced onion
- 2 Tbsp minced jalapeño pepper
  Juice of 1 lemon
- 2 oz tortilla chips

Combine the cilantro and garlic on a cutting board and use the back of a chef's knife to work them into a fine paste; a pinch of coarse salt helps this process. (If you own a mortar and pestle, there's never been a better time to use it.) Transfer the paste to a bowl and add the avocado. Use a fork to smash the avocado into a mostly smooth—but still slightly chunky—puree. Stir in the onion, jalapeño, lemon juice, and salt. Serve with tortilla chips or warm corn tortillas.

4 SERVINGS

190
CALORIES

14
G FAT

2
G SAT. FAT

357
MG SODIUM

6
G FIBER

*Always buy Hass, or California, avocados—the ones with the dark pebbly skin. They have a higher healthy fat content and creamier taste and texture.

Pico de Gallo

The most versatile of all salsas, this chunky mix of fresh produce can be scattered on tacos or nachos, folded into eggs and salads, strewn on sandwiches, or eaten with a batch of homemade tortilla chips. You really can't lose.

6 SERVINGS

15 CALORIES

0 G FAT

0 G SAT. FAT

100 MG SODIUM

1 G FIBER

- 4 Roma tomatoes, chopped
- 1 small red onion, diced
- 1 jalapeño, minced
- 1 handful cilantro, chopped
  Juice of 1 lime
  Salt and pepper to taste

Combine the tomatoes, onion, jalapeño, cilantro, and lime juice in a mixing bowl. Season with salt and pepper and mix to combine thoroughly. Keeps covered in the refrigerator for up to 1 week.

Spice Roasted Nuts

Toasting nuts awakens and deepens their natural flavor, plus it allows you to customize them with your own favorite spice mixtures. Here are four reliable routes to take.

4 SERVINGS

FOR CHILI ALMONDS

⅛ tsp chili powder + ⅛ tsp cayenne pepper + salt + 1 cup whole unpeeled almonds
116 CALORIES   **11** G FAT   **2** G SAT. FAT   **20** MG SODIUM   **2** G FIBER

FOR CURRIED CASHEWS

1 tsp curry powder + 1 cup unsalted cashews
111 CALORIES   **9** G FAT   **2** G SAT. FAT   **3** MG SODIUM   **1** G FIBER

FOR FIVE-SPICE PEANUTS

½ tsp Chinese five-spice powder + 1 cup salted peanuts

120 CALORIES   **11** G FAT   **2** G SAT. FAT   **11** MG SODIUM   **1** G FIBER

FOR COCOA PECANS

½ Tbsp cocoa powder + ¼ tsp ground cinnamon + 2 Tbsp sugar + 1 cup pecan halves

128 CALORIES   **12** G FAT   **2** G SAT. FAT   **150** MG SODIUM   **1** G FIBER

Preheat the oven to 400°F. Heat 1 tablespoon butter and the appropriate spices in a small saucepan. Stir in the nuts, then spread them on a baking sheet. Roast for 10 to 12 minutes, until very fragrant and warm, but not overly toasted.

Smoky Deviled Eggs

It might not be the healthiest way to eat an egg (that honor would go to boiling or poaching), but in terms of snacks and finger foods, it's hard to beat this Southern speciality.

8	eggs
¼	cup olive-oil mayonnaise
½	Tbsp Dijon mustard
2	tsp canned chipotle pepper
	Salt and black pepper to taste
	Paprika (preferably the smoked Spanish-style paprika called pimenton*)
2	strips bacon, cooked and finely crumbled

4 SERVINGS

215 CALORIES

18 G FAT

5 G SAT. FAT

472 MG SODIUM

0 G FIBER

*Spanish-style paprika adds more than just a visual pop: It brings a smoky note to the eggs that reinforces the smoke from the bacon and the chipotle.

Bring a pot or large saucepan of water to a full boil. Carefully lower the eggs into the water and cook for 8 minutes. Drain and immediately place in a bowl of ice water. When the eggs have cooled, peel them while still in the water (the water helps the shell slide off).

Cut the eggs in half and scoop out the yolks. Combine the yolks with the mayo, mustard, chipotle, and a good pinch of salt and pepper. Stir to combine thoroughly. Scoop the mixture into a sealable plastic bag, pushing it all the way into one corner. Cut a small hole in the corner. Squeeze to pipe the yolk mixture back into the whites. Top each with a sprinkle of paprika and a bit of crumbled bacon.

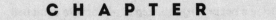

CHAPTER

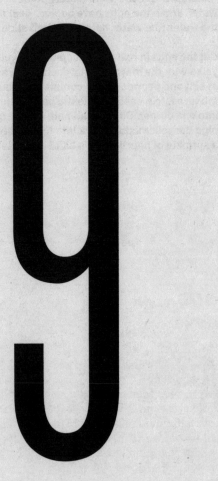

THE 8-HOUR DIET

Change Your Mind to Change Your Body

Seize control of your food cravings

and start enjoying your meals

As a health editor and former fat kid, I have tried dozens of diets.

Now, don't label me some sort of fad follower. I know from more than 20 years of health and fitness research that most diets work in the short term, but almost all fail in the long term, because they rely for the most part on willpower and gimmicks. Still, it's always been important to understand what the latest trends are, even while holding onto my healthy skepticism.

I've gone low carb, low fat, gluten free, meat free, even solid-food free. If there were a nothing-but-blueberry-pie diet out there, I would have turned into that kid from Willy Wonka's Chocolate Factory by now. Which is part of the reason I'm so excited about the 8-Hour Diet: It's the first diet plan ever devised in which you don't have to give up anything.

In fact, I have never appreciated food more—or indulged as freely in it—as I do now. Partly it's because the 8-Hour Diet allows me to eat whatever I want, as much as I want. I can seek out the creamiest ice cream, the juiciest steaks, the tangiest barbecue ribs, the cheesiest mac & cheese. I eat the food I love, I love the food I eat, and I eat as much as I want.

Slimmer and Stress Free!

Something else happened when I began to eat according to the principles of the 8-Hour Diet. The food I ate tasted better. I was no longer grazing mindlessly; instead, I was eating mindfully. I focused on choosing food I really wanted to eat and enjoying each meal and snack. It was like going from listening to a scratchy transistor radio to having digital surround sound.

Maybe that's why eating the 8-Hour Diet way has been popular with the great minds of the last many millennia. The scientific evidence for this diet is new, but wiser men than me have been following a similar type of eating for eons. The Big Four of religion—Moses, Jesus, Buddha, and Muhammad—all practiced and promoted fasting, and chances are they knew a thing or two more than we do. And while I'm not recommending 40 days and nights in the desert (at least not until they open a decent Starbucks in the Sinai), the health benefits of giving your body a longer break between meals are undeniable. Smart people through history, from Socrates to Hippocrates to Gandhi, found strength in skipping meals.

And they weren't doing it so they could get six-pack abs. "Fasting is known to be associated with psychological effects—peace and tranquillity," says Ron Evans, PhD, the researcher from the Salk Institute. "In fact, crime rates decrease during Ramadan [the Islamic fasting month]." He attributes this tranquil effect to "better stabilization of blood glucose during fasting."

James B. Johnson, MD, at Louisiana State University, has tested hundreds of patients who fast every other day. "Alternate-day dieters describe an improvement in mood," he says. "They often describe this feeling as wired, euphoric, like being in love, or like the Energizer Bunny."

So add to a leaner body and a longer life the delicious side effect of tranquillity and lower stress. And as long as you do your best to eat your 8-Hour Powerfoods each day, you'll know you're maximizing your nutritional intake, so both your mind and your body can function at their highest levels while keeping you in peak health.

Never Feel Hungry

That said, there are a lot of reasons for eating that go beyond simple nutrition. We eat to celebrate. We eat to mourn. We eat because we want comfort. We eat because we're bored. We eat because we're worried whether Iron Man, Thor, and the Hulk can stop the evil forces of Loki. And sometimes we eat just because it's there.

In fact, if there's one small hitch in the 8-Hour Diet, it's the fact that we all have the tendency to pick up food mindlessly and put it in our mouths. And let's get real, Moses: It's a lot easier to fast when you're up on a desert mountain with a Burning Bush than it is when you're down at the county mall with a Bob's Big Boy.

Fortunately, there's plenty of room for cheating in this plan. Following the plan just 3 days a week will work wonders on your belly. But on those days when you're trying to stick to the principles of the 8-Hour Diet, it helps to have some stamina-strengthening strategies, especially when the sweet scent of Cinnabon sends its fragrant aromas up your nose.

To help you repel the need to nosh, I tapped the genius brain trusts at *Men's Health, Women's Health,* and *Prevention* magazines for the very best, scientifically proven techniques for winning the mind-over-munchies battle. And it turns out there's a ton of research on the subject. These tips were so ingenious and so useful to me as I followed this program that I resolved to offer them to you, as well.

My purpose here isn't to weigh you down with 100 new items for your to-do list. Nobody, including me, uses all of these strategies. (I do have my favorites, though; especially tips 2, 7, 12, 21, 41, 57, 91, 95 to 97, and 100. Which do you like best?) But when Betsy in Accounting brings in a doughnut tray to the office tomorrow morning, or when Jon Stewart's punch lines are punctuated by pizza ads tomorrow night, don't let it get to you. Look here instead.

This list can help you in two ways.

FIRST: Distraction always works. Have you ever sat through a speech and noticed, as the speaker drones on and the air goes out of the room, more and more people in the audience suddenly feel the need to cough? Is it because people have allergic reactions to public presentations? No, it's boredom. When the mind has nothing to occupy it, the body takes over, trying to make things interesting. It's one of the reasons we eat when we're bored. If you can divert your mind from focusing on food, you win the battle every time.

SECOND: It helps to keep your mouth busy. Often the solution for wanting something to eat is having something to drink. The same area of the brain that controls hunger—the hypothalamus—also controls thirst. So if you're feeling a tickle to eat, start by just drinking instead. Peppermint tea. Black tea. Ice water with lemon. Iced tea. Sparkling water with crushed mint leaves. The quaffing possibilities are endless, but what you need to know now is this: If you're tempted to sup, you can often sip just as happily.

This list is built on proven appetite science, along with sneaky psychological tricks, that can see you through the most alluring temptations. To change your waistline, just learn to change the subject. And suddenly, it will be all about how you look and not about what you eat. It's time to take charge of both.

100 WAYS TO CUT OUT THE CALORIES

1 WATCH A FUNNY YOUTUBE VIDEO. Scientists in Brazil say that laughter may really be the best medicine—activating your "happy hormone" serotonin could reduce appetite.

2 THAT UPCOMING PROJECT DEADLINE YOU'VE BEEN PUTTING OFF? Git 'r done. When procrastinators grow anxious or bored, they're more likely to give in to their impulses (like feeding a growling stomach) to improve their mood, according to a study published in the *Journal of Personality and Social Psychology*.

3 MAKE A PLAN TO KNOCK OUT HUNGER. Dutch researchers report that dieters who wrote a list of "if-then" statements were more successful in attaining goals. For example: "If I get hungry at noon, then I'll spend my lunch hour at the gym."

4 WHEN A CRAVING STRIKES, MAKE A FIST. In a study published in the *Journal of Consumer Research,* people who tightened their muscles (regardless of which ones) while trying to exert self-control in their food choices were better able to overcome temptations. Our mind-body connection associates firm muscles with firm willpower.

5 IMAGINE YOURSELF BITING INTO A BIG, JUICY BURGER. A Carnegie Mellon University study found that simply visualizing yourself eating a certain food kick-starts a psychological effect called *habituation*—and your motivation to actually eat the food decreases.

6 WHEN THE THREAT OF MUNCHIES REARS ITS UGLY HEAD, CALL YOUR MOM. Hearing a supportive, familiar voice prompts the brain to release oxytocin, a stress-fighting, mood-elevating hormone, according to a study from the University of Wisconsin–Madison. Reducing stress is linked to increases in your satiety hormone, leptin.

7 THROW AWAY YOUR DESKTOP SNACKS AND AVOID THE CAFETERIA. The sight and smell of food can cause the body to experience hunger, whether or not you actually have an appetite.

8 JUST BREATHE. Deep breathing can stimulate the production of insulin, which lowers blood sugar levels. While you're slowly inhaling and exhaling, repeat a short phrase or song lyric to yourself to help stay focused.

9 COVER YOUR DESK WITH A BLACK TABLECLOTH DURING THE DAY OR CHANGE YOUR COMPUTER BACKGROUND TO BLACK. According to the book *Prescription for Nutritional Healing,* the color black may naturally suppress your appetite. Violet works as well—but we'll leave that one up to you.

10 READ A THRILLER. Getting caught up in a good story will distract you from thoughts of food.

11 FLIP THROUGH OLD PHOTO ALBUMS—PREFER-ABLY, ONES OF YOU AT YOUR PHYSICAL PEAK THAT BRING TO MIND HAPPIER TIMES. Not only will this give you a weight-loss goal, but researchers from the University of Southampton found that feeling nostalgic increases self-regard, social bonds, and positive feelings—all things that will leave you psychologically primed for 8-Hour Diet success.

12 WORK ON YOUR KILL/DEATH RATIO. Stanford researchers found that playing video games stimulates the brain's reward system—the part of the brain that might long for the excitement normally provided by food.

13 KEEP AN 8-HOUR DIET JOURNAL. Like a food journal, sans food. Make detailed notes about your thoughts, feelings, and physical reactions, then reread them to reflect on your experience, lock in success strategies, and marvel at your progress.

14 FIND YOUR MANTRA. If you're tempted to break your food schedule, remind yourself why you started this plan in the first place and repeat that thought over to yourself until the temptation subsides.

15 WHEN YOU START TO FEEL A FOOD CRAVING, HIT THE STOPWATCH ON YOUR CELL PHONE. Record the time it takes for your crave to fade, and use it to count down your next pang.

16 USE YOUR IMAGINATION. Sports psychologists tell us that when people visualize themselves doing something, it's more likely to happen. Picture a coworker enticing you with fresh baked goods and see yourself standing firm. This prepares you to deal with temptation.

17 **DON'T WASTE YOUR WILLPOWER.** You have a finite store of this cognitive currency, according to a Case Western Reserve University study. So rid yourself of problem situations that will use it up—make decisions and stick with them, delegate headaches, quit procrastinating—to preserve your will for when you really need it. With Chicago-style pizza and beer with the gang, for instance.

18 **PLAY "WORDS WITH FRIENDS" WITH LOTS OF FRIENDS (ESPECIALLY SMART ONES).** You're less likely to dwell on your hunger when your brain is busy figuring out how to use Q, A, and T (tropical plant used as a stimulant). Really, any word game will do—on a game board, online, or on your smartphone.

19 **CLUE IN A FRIEND.** Social support and interpersonal pressure can help with self-control, so explain the 8-Hour Diet to a friend and ask her to check in on you to see how you're doing.

20 **MAKE YOUR BED.** Your brain is a creature of habit—and having a routine can build willpower and discipline. Try something simple, like flossing every day or reading before bed; this will increase the likelihood of your following through on other healthy habits as well.

21 **FIND INSPIRATION IN OTHER 8-HOUR DIETERS.** Read success stories in this book or online for a little extra motivation, and think to yourself, "If she could do it, so can I!"

22 **DON'T BE A REFRIGERATOR STALKER.** Put a note on the fridge door to eliminate the unconscious habit of repeatedly opening it. It's the doorway to trouble, and you don't want to go there.

23 GO GREEN—WITH TEA, THAT IS. Green tea suppresses appetite and can aid in fat burning. Opt for an organic, caffeinated option to keep you going throughout the day.

24 FOLLOW THE LEAD OF OUR ANCESTORS. When you feel intimidated, remind yourself that our ancestors often went days without food. It's a challenge, but you can do it.

25 SWITCH FROM YOUR JEANS AND T-SHIRT TO SOMETHING SNAZZIER. Wearing business casual attire makes workers feel more authoritative, productive, and competent than everyday casual, according to a study from the University of Southern Indiana. Giving yourself a confidence boost can translate to greater confidence in your ability to stick with the diet.

26 CHECK YOUR CHECKLIST. Write a list of all the specific reasons why your fast will help you. Reflecting on these things will help at times when your motivation is running low.

27 SIP YOUR WAY TO SATIETY. You've heard it a million times—for good reason. Water is the most natural, inexpensive, and effective appetite suppressant around. Drink it.

28 PREPARE A CUP OF PEPPERMINT TEA. It can help fight cravings, improve digestion, and even alleviate headaches.

29 ADD A LITTLE ZEST TO MAKE YOUR WATER A LITTLE MORE SATISFYING. Squeeze sliced oranges, lemons, or limes into your glass for a boost of antioxidants that can temper your hunger.

30 KEEP YOURSELF SIPPING WITH GREAT-TASTING WATER. Let a pitcher of room-temperature water with sprigs of mint or lemongrass sit overnight so the flavors set. Both herbs have health benefits such as aiding digestion and relieving headaches.

31 SET A GOAL, AND THEN NAIL IT. A 2006 study found that people who set goals were less anxious and felt better about themselves than their less goal-oriented counterparts. Make it short term—like drinking at least 3 cups of green tea during your 16-hour food break.

32 LEARN TO LOVE OOLONG. The tea fights cancer, burns fat, and is packed with antioxidants. Brew a cup 1 hour before you work out—studies have shown an increase in energy expenditure and 12 percent higher fat oxidation associated with the drink.

33 TAKE ON THE NEW CINNAMON CHALLENGE. Add a teaspoon of cinnamon to your tea every day. A Chinese study found that cinnamon regulates blood pressure levels and delays the passing of food (or tea) from the stomach into the intestine, making you feel fuller longer.

34 WAKE UP WITH YERBA MATÉ. This South American drink gives you the same vitality and alertness as coffee but without the jitters, and it acts as an appetite suppressant to curb hunger.

35 ADD SOME SPARKLE TO YOUR DRINK. When hunger pangs strike, drink a glass of seltzer water with lime for taste. Those gassy bubbles fill you up more than non-sparkling water.

36 TAKE A URINE TEST. If your urine is darker than light straw, you may not be drinking enough fluid. Check the color, and then bottoms up.

37 WALK TO A WATER FOUNTAIN—THE ONE ON THE OTHER SIDE OF YOUR OFFICE. Frequent, short breaks to fill your glass provide a quick energy lift. Just a few minutes of brisk activity makes your heart pump and your lungs expand, increasing oxygen flow throughout the body and stimulating brain chemicals to shed fatigue.

38 PLAN YOUR OWN ICE CAPADES. Simply chop up your additive of choice (cucumber or mint works well), add it to your ice-cube tray with water, and freeze. Sprucing things up is a sure way to enjoy your eight glasses.

39 BEAT HUNGER (AND DIABETES!) with black tea. A study in the *Journal of the American College of Nutrition* found that black tea decreases blood sugar levels by 10 percent for 2½ hours, so you'll feel fuller and avoid hunger later.

40 SIT DOWN WITH JOE. Although green tea may have more health benefits, caffeine in general has been shown to slightly reduce appetite. Especially if you're feeling fatigued later in the morning, hit the coffeepot.

41 HIT THE ROAD. Set a timer for 30 minutes and hit the road running. Just a half hour of hard running can reduce appetite by 50 percent for up to 2 hours, according to scientists at Loughborough University. Running increases production of peptide YY (an appetite suppressant) and reduces ghrelin (an appetite stimulant), and the jarring motion disturbs the digestive tract, quieting the impulse to eat.

42 OR HIT THE GYM. The study also found that strength training reduces ghrelin production by up to 25 percent. And the muscle you build will boost your metabolism.

43 MAKE YOUR OWN VEGETABLE STOCK. Simmer onions, carrots, celery, garlic, and one bay leaf in water for an hour. Drain and store in your refrigerator; pop a cupful in the microwave for a minute or two for a warm treat during the day.

44 **FIND A QUIET PLACE TO GRAB A FEW ZZZS.** People who are sleep deprived have higher levels of the hormone ghrelin, which tells your brain when you're hungry. Just 15 to 20 minutes is enough to reenergize you without affecting your ability to sleep at night.

45 **DO 15 MINUTES OF CHAIR-BASED YOGA.** It can curb work stress by reducing sympathetic nervous system activity. Scientists at the Fred Hutchinson Cancer Research Center found that people who practiced yoga had smaller appetites and more controlled eating habits. Start by lifting your arms above your head, and slowly bend to each side for 30 seconds.

46 **START A PICK-UP GAME AFTER WORK.** Exercise doesn't have to be boring—relive your glory days by challenging coworkers to a game of hoops or soccer.

47 **SPEND MORE TIME WITH YOUR PET.** Not only will it keep you moving and busy, but studies have shown that pet owners have significantly fewer stress-related increases in blood pressure. Stress and appetite are closely linked.

48 **OCCUPY YOUR HANDS AND YOUR TIME BY WOODWORKING OR WASHING YOUR CAR.** It's hard to visualize the food-to-mouth motion while your hands are covered in sawdust or soap.

49 **DO A 1-MINUTE BLITZ.** Pick an exercise (burpees, pushups, squat jumps, whatever) and see how many you can do in 1 minute. Trust us, your mind will be more focused on the burning in your legs than any faint hint of hunger. Any of the exercises in the 8-Minute Workout Chapter would be good here, too.

50 **STRETCH IT OUT.** Stationary stretching will warm your muscles without burning extra energy and it will help you shed stress and feel calmer.

51 **GO ON A BIKE RIDE OR CYCLE AT THE GYM.** A Surrey University study in England found that an hour of biking helps reduce your appetite by signaling an increase in appetite-suppressing hormones.

52 **TAKE A YOGA CLASS.** Studies have shown that yoga improves levels of serotonin—the molecule of will-power that, if kept at too low a level, can mean being unable to control your impulses.

53 **SET A POP-UP TIMER ON YOUR COMPUTER SO YOU GET OUT OF YOUR CHAIR.** Research from the University of Massachusetts revealed that the more you sit, the greater your appetite (sedentary subjects felt 17 percent hungrier than those who moved about throughout the day).

54 **FIND A NEW HOBBY TO KEEP BUSY.** Just make it something that's not an extension of your work life, to find balance. If you're a numbers cruncher, try something creative like learning a musical instrument. If your job is high-tech, try gardening or bird-watching.

55 **TRAIN IN INTERVALS.** Alternating full-force cardio with short rest periods will maximize your calorie burn and reduce levels of ghrelin, your hunger hormone.

56 **WALK AWAY.** Your hunger hormones spike when you're feeling frazzled, so turn off your phone and leave the stressful environment—even if just for a minute. You'll return feeling less overwhelmed and have less risk of being overfed.

57 **VOW TO WALK TO YOUR COWORKERS INSTEAD OF E-MAILING THEM.** Researchers at the University of Missouri found that every consecutive day of inactivity significantly increases blood sugar levels—26 percent, on average. Leaving your chair for just a minute throughout the day can help bring those levels back down.

58 **STIMULATE YOUR SENSES.** Dark chocolate suppresses appetite—but stick to the aroma. A 2010 study published in *Regulatory Peptides* found that smelling rather than eating the bitter candy is more effective at reducing levels of ghrelin, a hormone that stimulates hunger.

59 **CHEW A PIECE OF SUGAR-FREE GUM.** A University of Rhode Island study found that chewing stimulates nerves in the jaw that are connected to the area of the brain responsible for satiety. Males in particular felt less hungry and more energetic after popping a piece of sugarless.

60 **CHEW ICE.** Gnawing on ice when you get hungry will trick your brain into thinking you've eaten.

61 **BURN AWAY STOMACH GROWLING.** Light up candles scented with peppermint, banana, green apple, and vanilla. Studies have found that these fragrances in particular can trick your brain into thinking you've eaten.

62 **IF YOU'RE HITTING A WALL, PUT ON AN UPBEAT RADIO STATION.** Listening to music for about an hour a day can help reduce fatigue, according to a recent study. This will also boost your mood, so "emotional eating" won't set you back.

63 **LET THE SUN SHINE IN.** Stress causes your body to pump out cortisol, which creates a resistance to leptin— the satiety hormone. Just 10 minutes in the sun can make a tremendous difference in your stress level and give you a surge of energy.

64 **USE MEDITATION TECHNIQUES TO RELAX AND DIVERT YOUR ATTENTION.** Sit up straight in a quiet room, close your eyes, and concentrate on nothing but your breathing for 15 minutes. If you can't focus that long, start with 5-minute sessions and work your way up.

65 BRUSH YOUR TEETH, FLOSS, AND TOP IT OFF WITH MOUTHWASH. You're accustomed to thinking food tastes bad after brushing, so the fresh, minty taste will get your mind off eating.

66 CLEAN THE TOILET. Okay, maybe it sounds unpleasant, but hey, we bet your desire to eat will be flushed.

67 TURN DOWN THE AC. A study published in *Physiology & Behavior* found that exposure to temperatures above the "thermoneutral comfort zone" decreases appetite and food intake.

68 CUDDLE UP WITH YOUR SIGNIFICANT OTHER. Your brain releases the "love hormone," oxytocin, whenever you touch someone or feel loved. High levels can beat back stress and lower blood pressure. That sense of calm and appreciation will keep you from seeking other rewards—like the kind at the bottom of the cookie box.

69 SCHEDULE A MASSAGE. In one study, a 15-minute chair massage decreased hospital workers' cortisol levels by 24 percent. Cortisol can mix up your hunger signals and suppress your brain's normal reward system.

70 FIND RELEASE IN YOUR SECOND STRONGEST BODILY HUNGER: SEX. Oxytocin peaks in your body after climax. Less cortisol leads to fewer stomach growls. So, is your partner supportive of your weight-loss goals, or not?

71 WHILE YOUR BODY REBUILDS INSIDE, GIVE YOUR OUTSIDE SOME TLC. Go to the spa, have a facial, or reward yourself with an expensive moisturizer. Soothe yourself, calm your appetite.

72 SAY THANKS. Write a letter to someone who influenced your life in a positive way. Showing gratitude will counteract negative emotions and leave you feeling happier. Life satisfaction trumps patting a round belly—or stuffing one.

73 BUILD A FENCE OR LEARN TO PLAY A NEW SONG. Tasks that give you a sense of mastery can activate your brain's reward system, but make sure you're working toward a tangible goal. You'll be relaxed and completely immersed in nailing the right chord, leaving no time for food thoughts.

74 HOST A COUPLES' GAME NIGHT. Studies show that mutual cooperation is immediately rewarding (regardless of whether or not you win) because it enhances activity in brain circuits and boosts serotonin.

75 CLEAN OUT YOUR IN-BOX. How great is it when you can distract yourself from eating and accomplish something? Sift through e-mails and unsubscribe to those newsletters you never read—which make up an estimated 30 percent of the average in-box, according to a study by MessageGate.

76 PLAY YOUR PUP'S FAVORITE GAME—FRISBEE. This keeps your hands activated and provides some face time with your dog, friend, or partner. Busy life, busy hands, less stray time in front of the refrigerator. (Bonus points: Playing Ultimate Frisbee for 30 minutes can burn 330 calories.)

77 PARTNER UP AND DO THE DISHES. Anything to keep your mind and hands occupied is a hunger suppressor, and, according to a Pew Research Center survey, sharing chores ups your odds of having a happy marriage. (It's ranked third in importance, after faithfulness and a healthy sex life.)

78 MAKE AMENDS. If you had a recent falling-out with someone, write him or her a letter to patch things up. In a study published in the *Journal of Obesity,* participants who focused on forgiveness toward others experienced an increase in mindfulness, reduced anxiety, and less likelihood of eating in response to food cues.

79 MAKE A LIST OF WHAT KILLED YOUR RELATIVES. It may sound a little morbid, but it'll give you a heads-up on ailments you may be at risk of, as well as motivate you to keep up your healthy choices.

80 SPEND 15 MINUTES TALKING TO A COWORKER. Even if they're glancing at the clock, you're staying distracted and improving your health. Plus, you won't talk with your mouth full, right? According to a Tel Aviv University study, those who have good relationships with coworkers live longer.

81 TRY LIGHT THERAPY. Low levels of serotonin are often associated with cravings, specifically for carbs. Boost your happy hormone by keeping a bright light at your desk or seeking sunlight as the day (and your willpower) wears on.

82 KILL CRAVINGS WITH KINDNESS. Help a neighbor carry in groceries or give a coworker a compliment; try to commit random acts of kindness whenever possible. In a study published in the *Journal of Obesity,* participants who used loving-kindness techniques in their mindfulness practice showed reduced frequency of emotional eating.

83 VISUALIZE YOURSELF RUNNING ON THE BEACH—OR WHATEVER IT IS YOU CAN'T WAIT TO DO WHEN YOU'RE AT YOUR GOAL WEIGHT. Play out the entire scene in your mind, including all your senses to make it a whole-brain experience. Being immersed in this play-by-play will connect you with your reasons for dieting, according to ThinWithin.com.

84 **GO FOR A SPIN.** Literally. Stand up and twirl five times, or up to 20 times, then take a 1-minute break and do it again. Keep your eyes fixed at a spot on the wall while spinning to avoid dizziness. When your brain is busy reestablishing equilibrium, it might forget your food crush on chocolate chip cookies. (Temporarily, at least; maybe the cookie tray will be empty by the time your brain recovers.)

85 **ADD SOME POTPOURRI TO YOUR OFFICE.** A recent study found that jasmine scent has specific hunger-killing powers and can also reduce anxiety and boost energy. Store the potpourri in a drawer and pull it out in case of food emergencies.

86 **CLOSE YOUR EYES, BREATHE IN THROUGH YOUR NOSE, OUT THROUGH YOUR MOUTH, AND VIVIDLY IMAGINE YOURSELF DOING YOUR FAVORITE THING.** Think about what you would wear, see, smell, and feel. Scientists at McGill University in Montreal tested this "pleasant imagery method" and found it curbed cravings in everyday life.

87 **WATCH TRAFFIC ON THE HIGHWAY OR TENNIS ON TV OR YOUR KIDS PLAYING PING-PONG.** The back-and-forth eye movements may help you forget food thoughts. One study found that visually tracking a rapidly moving stimulus reduces the intensity of food images in the brain.

88 **TRY FOREHEAD TRACKING, A TECHNIQUE PROVEN TO REDUCE FOOD THOUGHTS AND CRAVINGS.** Tap an imaginary line with your finger from temple to temple: one tap per second, 1 centimeter at a time. Follow your finger with your eyes, focusing on the first joint in your pointer. This occupies the limited-capacity visual region of your brain and crowds out yearnings for Yoo-hoo.

89 **LEARN THE ANCIENT ART OF TAI CHI, A FORM OF CHINESE MARTIAL ARTS THAT COMBINES SLOW MOVEMENTS WITH MEDITATION AND BREATHING TO CALM YOUR BODY AND MIND.** It can burn as many calories as moderate-intensity activities, such as walking. Focusing on learning a new physical skill that involves the mind will distract you from any other annoying, recurring thoughts.

90 **TAKE A BEATING.** Studies show that people with high heart-rate variability—moment-by-moment fluctuations in heart rhythm—have more self-control, and deep breathing can boost it. Try this Hindu breathing technique called *ujjayi:* Inhale through your nose for 6 seconds, then exhale through your mouth for 6 seconds, like you're trying to fog up a mirror. Next, try doing the same thing just through your nose, while making a rushing sound in the back of your throat.

91 **LEND A HELPING HAND.** Take an hour out of your day (your lunch hour, perhaps) to volunteer in your town. One study shows that just thinking about doing something generous releases happy hormones serotonin and dopamine, so you won't rely on a Twinkie to trigger them instead.

92 **TAP INTO YOUR SPIRITUALITY.** Religious fasting, such as the Islamic month of Ramadan, places huge emphasis on prayer during the process. Pray at home or go to church. University of Mississippi researchers found that churchgoers had lower levels of stress hormones, on average, than those who did not attend services at all. What's more, according to research from Tel Aviv University, ritualistic-like repetitive behaviors (such as praying) induce calm and give a heightened sense of control—which may come in handy in showing your cravings who's boss.

93 **GO GREEN TO STAY FOCUSED.** Place an English ivy plant on your desk and you'll concentrate on your work rather than get sidetracked by food thoughts. The reason: Leafy green plants absorb benzene emitted by office supplies, which can disrupt the central nervous system, slow thinking, and break concentration. And when your mind wanders, we know what trouble it can get into.

94 LOCK FINGERS WITH YOUR ONE-AND-ONLY.
Holding hands reduces stress-related activity in the brain's hypothalamus, the seat of your feelings for hunger and thirst. Holding hands also lowers those hunger-stoking cortisol levels and calms the part of the brain that registers pain, which can keep you from feeling it as much.

95–97 BE YOUR OWN ACUPRESSURIST (NO NEEDLES!).
According to the Chinese therapeutic system, energy meridians run along your body, correlating to main organ systems. By massaging these meridians, you can stimulate these organs when they're deficient in energy, says Dr. Christina Winsey, DC, founder of TheICanDoctor .com. Gently rub each of these three appetite-control acupressure points for several minutes when you're having hunger pangs.

Jaw: Put your index fingers in front of the fleshy part of both ears (the part you usually push to drown out sound). If you can feel your jaw move when you open your mouth, you've found it.

Earlobe: Beneath where the lobe connects with your face is another hunger-relieving point.

Crease of the knee: Find and massage the center point in the crease on the underside of your kneecap.

98 SIP WARM LEMON WATER.
Drinking lemon water can help ensure normal functioning of the circulatory system and keep skin hydrated, and some people find that it reduces appetite. The warm temperature is soothing and will help counteract your body's craving for comfort food when it's cold.

99 SCHEDULE MORE EXHILARATING EXERCISE, LIKE A MARTIAL ARTS CLASS, ROCK CLIMBING, OR MOUNTAIN BIKING. Physical activity, combined with a little risk taking, will make you look forward to your workout.

100 THE ALL-PURPOSE, ANYONE-CAN-FOLLOW-IT ÜBER TIP: DO ANYTHING FOR 15 MINUTES AT THE FIRST SIGN OF HUNGER PANGS TO GIVE THEM TIME TO WANE. Research shows that dips in blood sugar associated with hunger return to normal after 10 to 15 minutes. And that may be all that stands between you and success on the 8-Hour Diet!

CHAPTER

10

THE 8-HOUR DIET

The 8-Minute Workouts

Turbocharge the 8-Hour Diet
in just 8 minutes a day!

What? It's true. With just 8 minutes each day—plus a simple strategy of maximizing your calorie burn through nonexercise methods—you'll shed fat even faster.

There are certain things that just seem too good to be real: Mark McGwire's home run record. Jenny McCarthy's décolletage. Tony Bennett's hair.

And right up there with those suspicious phenomena? A workout lasting just 8 minutes a day.

I know, I know: Everyone from the US government to the unemployed actor masquerading as a trainer at your gym has told you that you need *at least* 30 to 40 minutes three times a week, at minimum, for optimum health and weight management. The entire idea of an 8-minute workout goes against all the prevailing wisdom.

And that's true—unless you're following the 8-Hour Diet, in which case 8 minutes is all you need.

Here's why: Unlike the average American who's feasting 24/7, you've started an eating program that gives your body's energy centers—the mitochondria—a break from processing food. And you've begun training your body to burn its own fat for energy. Each day that you follow the 8-Hour Diet, you melt a little more unwanted flab, simply by going about your day. But when you jump-start your day with a tiny bit of exercise, you tap into your fat stores earlier and more effectively, so you melt even more fat.

Mark Mattson, PhD, of the National Institute for Aging, believes that eating for only a limited time each day and adding in exercise is the most powerful fat-fighting tool ever discovered. "There's a lot of evidence in bodybuilders that it's best to exercise at the end of a period when you haven't eaten," he says. "It's better for building muscle." And if I've learned anything as a health editor, it's that muscle is more metabolically active than fat. The more muscle you have, the more calories your body burns, and the leaner you grow. So fasting, added to exercise, means you're combusting the maximum possible energy and losing the most weight you possibly can. Good job!

Dr. Mattson goes on: "When you haven't eaten for a while, the muscle cells enhance their ability to take up glucose, so their insulin sensitivity increases as well as their ability to take up amino acids. Then you exercise, which puts more of an acute stress on the muscle cells. The cells are highly primed to pick up energy and amino acids and to grow and rebuild muscle proteins." In this case, "growing muscle" does not equal looking like the Incredible Hulk when he's having a bad day, but rather it means the lean, shapely muscle that makes a woman (and a man) look fitter and healthier come swimsuit season.

But Dr. Mattson isn't finished piling up the benefits, and the next one will be music to your ears: "There will be more fat loss," he tells us. As you may have read in earlier chapters, much of the caloric value of the food you eat is stored in the liver as glycogen. By following the 8-Hour Diet and not running your liver the way Howard Stern runs his mouth (i.e., constantly), you give your body the chance to burn off that glycogen and start burning fat. And that happens regardless of whether you exercise or not—just going about your day will eventually burn off your glycogen stores and your body will begin tapping into the fat.

But if you add just a little exercise into the mix? By exercising before your first meal of the day, you hasten the glycogen burn—and maximize the amount of time your body is burning fat.

Now, does it make sense to exercise for more than 8 minutes? Sure, if you want. But it's more important to get into a habit of consistency and make physical movement a part of as many days a week as possible. To help you along, I borrowed the minds of some of the best exercise experts in the world and channeled them through the expertise of the *Men's Health* fitness team.

Some of what follows will be challenging, but there are supereasy workouts here as well—starting with a simple 8-minute walk. Will walking 8 minutes a day give you abs like Ryan Lochte? No, but you're not looking to burn 1,000 calories, or even 100 necessarily. You're looking to boost your metabolism in order to tap into your glycogen stores. Combined with the 8-Hour Diet, even this easy bit of movement will ignite your fat burners faster and speed you on the path to leanness. Then, work your way up to harder workouts. Combine them into 16-, 24-, or 32-minute workouts. But aim for consistency: I'd rather see you do 8 minutes a day than 32 minutes once or twice a week.

THE
8-MINUTE
WORKOUTS

ONE-EXERCISE ROUTINES

If you're not a regular exerciser, there's no need to rush into a strenuous new workout plan. A beginner's goal is just to burn a few extra calories to help your body deplete its glycogen stores.

Walking

EXERCISE

1

OPTION 1: Simply take a brisk walk for 8 minutes in the morning.

OPTION 2: Walk on a treadmill at a slight incline for 8 minutes. Increase the incline for a greater calorie burn.

NOTE: To turn this into a personal challenge, walk as far as you can, as fast as you can, for 4 minutes, then turn around and walk back. Aim to walk just a little bit farther each day—either by extending your time, or by upping your speed.

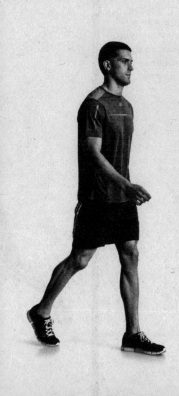

Running Outside

EXERCISE

2

NOTE: You can try this same routine on a stationary bike, rowing machine, or other aerobic equipment.

OPTION 1: Jog at a steady pace that allows you to talk, but only in short spurts of three or four words at a time.

OPTION 2: Go easy, go hard. Jog at a light, easy pace for 30 seconds. Then step up your pace a couple of notches for 30 seconds. Continue to repeat back and forth.

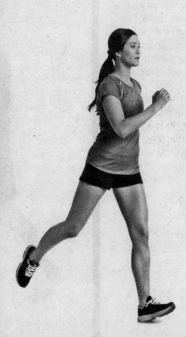

Running in Place

EXERCISE

3

MORE OPTIONS! Use this running in place routine in combination with jumping jacks, seal jacks, or jump rope.

Run in place for 60 seconds, trying to raise your knees high. Rest for 60 seconds. Run for another 60 seconds, and rest for 60 seconds. Then run for 60 seconds, only now move backward and forward a few feet as you do it. Rest for 60 seconds. Run for 60 seconds again, but as you do, move a few feet to the left and then a few feet back to the right. Rest for 30 seconds. Then finish up by running for 30 seconds in place.

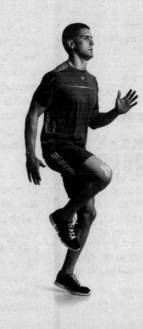

Burpees

EXERCISE

4

MAKE IT
EASIER

Instead of kicking your legs back simultaneously, slowly straighten one leg behind you, and then the other. Reverse the movement and then stand up.

MAKE IT
HARDER

Add a pushup each time you kick your legs back. Also, you can jump up from the squat position instead of simply standing.

Set a timer for 8 minutes. Your goal is to complete 8 rounds of a level in 8 minutes. For instance, in level 1 you will attempt 4 reps every minute for 8 minutes. Once you can do 8 rounds in 8 minutes, move on to the next level. Don't rush at first; focus on maintaining good form and building both strength and flexibility.

LEVEL	REPETITIONS
1	4
2	5
3	6
4	7
5	8
6	9

Stand in front of a low box (about 6 to 12 inches high) with your feet set wider than shoulder-width apart. Bending at your hips and knees, lower your body into a squat until you can place your palms on the box (1). Kick your legs backward (2), then reverse the move and pull your legs back to the squat position (3). Then quickly stand up (4). That's 1 rep.

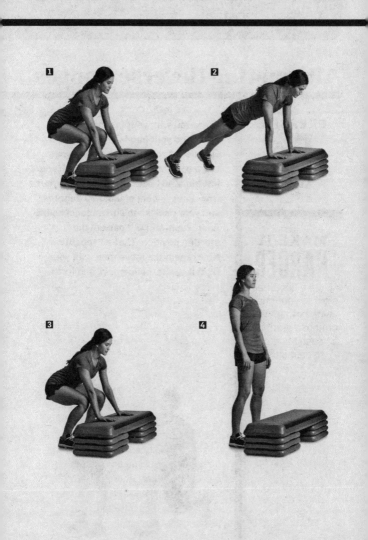

**TWO-EXERCISE
ROUTINES**

Here are three two-exercise routines that combine two toning exercises and can be done with just your body weight. They emphasize hard-to-tone areas like the

Alternating Reverse Lunges

EXERCISE

5a

Stand tall with your feet hip-width apart and your hands in front of your chest or at your sides. Keeping your torso upright, step backward with your left foot and lower your body until your front knee is bent at least 90 degrees and your back knee almost touches the floor. Push yourself back to the starting position. That's 1 repetition. Now repeat the movement with your right leg, alternating back and forth.

**MAKE IT
HARDER**

Hold a dumbbell next to your chest with both hands, or hold a dumbbell in each hand next to your sides.

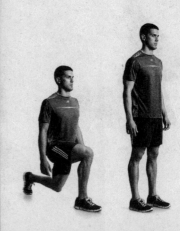

Mountain Climber

EXERCISE

5b

Assume a pushup position with your arms completely straight. Your body should form a straight line from your head to your ankles. Without allowing your lower-back posture to change, lift your right foot off the floor and slowly move your right knee toward your chest. Return to the starting position, and repeat with your left leg. Alternate back and forth for the duration of the set.

MAKE IT

EASIER

Place your hands on an elevated surface, such as a bench or ottoman.

MAKE IT

HARDER

Place your feet on an elevated surface, such as a bench or ottoman.

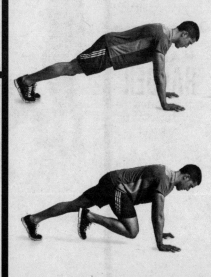

Body-Weight Power Squat

EXERCISE
6a

Stand with your feet slightly beyond shoulder-width apart, toes forward, hands next to your sides. Simultaneously push your hips back and swing your arms backward, lowering your body until your thighs are close to parallel to the floor. Pause, and then quickly push yourself back to the starting position as you swing your arms above your head, ending the movement on your toes.

MAKE IT
EASIER

Place a box or chair behind your body, and squat to the surface each repetition. Pause momentarily, then push yourself up.

MAKE IT
HARDER

Jump up from the down position of the squat.

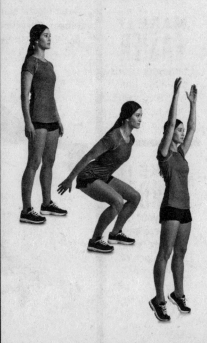

Bucking Hop

EXERCISE

6b

MAKE IT

HARDER

Increase the
height and
distance of each
hop.

Get down on all fours, with your hands
and knees on the floor. Now raise your
knees off the floor an inch or two.
Without changing the posture of your
lower back, "hop" your feet off the
floor and to the right. (Imagine there's
an imaginary line that you're hopping
over.) Then immediately hop to the left.
Continue hopping back and forth,
keeping your hips and shoulders
square throughout the exercise. The
key is to keep most of your weight on
your shoulders to allow a smooth
transfer from side to side.

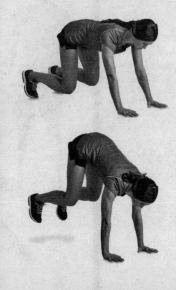

Alternating Lateral Lunge

EXERCISE

7a

Stand with your feet about hip-width apart. Take a big step to your left, lowering your body by pushing your hips back and bending your left knee until your thigh is close to parallel to the floor. (Don't let your right foot rise off the floor.) Return to the starting position, then repeat the movement to your right.

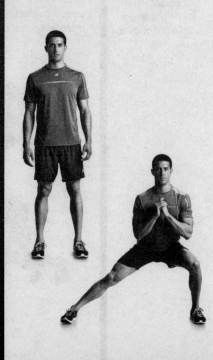

Pushup Hold with Knee-Elbow Touch

EXERCISE

7b

Assume a standard pushup position. Lift your right foot, bend your knee, and try to touch your knee to your right elbow. Return to the starting position and repeat with your left leg. That's 1 rep.

MAKE IT
HARDER

Do a pushup as you perform the knee-to-elbow touch, as shown in the bottom photograph.

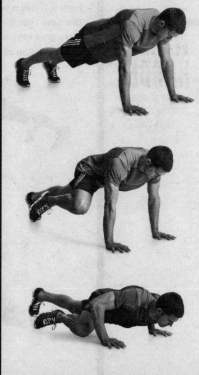

T-Rotation

EXERCISE

8a

MAKE IT
HARDER

Do a pushup between each rotation.

Assume a pushup position, your arms straight. In one movement, lift your right hand and rotate the right side of your body upward, until you're facing sideways. Your arms and body now form a T. Reverse the move and repeat, this time rotating your left side. Note: Keep your hips raised and your body in a straight line as you rotate.

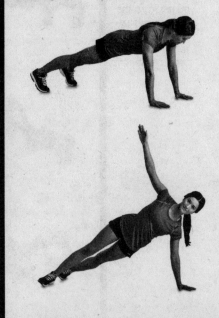

one round. Rest 1 minute. Do a second round, and rest for another 60 seconds. Then do your third round, and you're done—8 minutes of intense calorie burn.

Hip Extension

Lie on your back with your knees bent and feet flat. Place your arms at an angle out to your sides, palms down. Raise your hips so your body is straight from shoulders to knees. Pause for 1 to 2 seconds, lower your hips to the floor, and repeat.

MAKE IT
HARDER
Place your fingertips on your forehead.

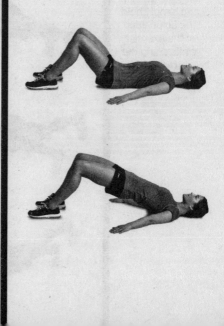

Pushup with Leg Lift

EXERCISE

9a

MAKE IT
EASIER

Skip the pushup
and simply hold
the up position
of the exercise
while doing the
alternating
leg lifts.

Assume a pushup position with your arms completely straight. Your body should form a straight line from your head to your ankles. Without allowing your hips to sag, lift your right foot off the floor and do a pushup. Return to the starting position, and repeat with your left leg. Alternate back and forth for the duration of the set.

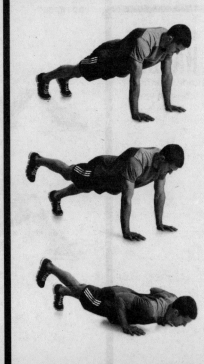

Body-Weight Rotational Squat

EXERCISE
9b

MAKE IT
HARDER
Increase the speed at which you perform the movement, while staying under control.

Stand with your feet beyond shoulder-width apart. Push your hips back and bend your knees to lower your body as far as you can without losing the natural arch of your spine. Now push yourself back to the starting position. As you rise up, pivot your feet and rotate your torso to the right. Reverse the movement, and then rotate to your left. Continue to alternate back and forth.

Judo Pushup

EXERCISE

10a

MAKE IT
EASIER

Simply move back and forth from the upside-down V position to the standard starting position of a pushup.

Begin in a pushup position but move your feet hip-width apart and forward, and raise your hips so your body almost forms an upside-down V. Lower the front of your body down and forward until your chin nears the floor. Then squeeze your glutes and lower your hips as you straighten your arms and raise your head and shoulders toward the ceiling. Now push your hips back up into the upside-down V and repeat.

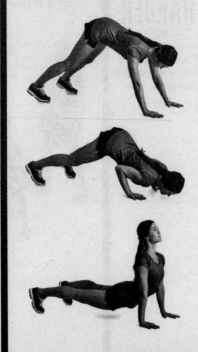

Duck Walk

EXERCISE

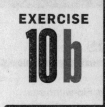

Stand with your feet hip-width apart and place your hands behind your head, flaring your elbows and squeezing your shoulder blades back and down. Squat as far down as you can and walk forward and backward without raising or lowering your hips.

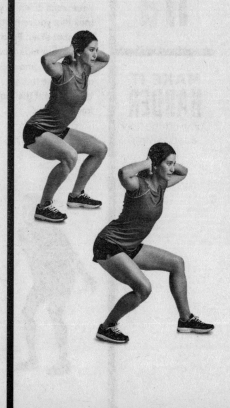

UP & AT 'EM
BLOOD
PUMPERS

These are fast-moving exercises that get
the blood flowing and the heart rate up. Do
one exercise for 20 seconds, and rest for

Ground Zero Jumps

EXERCISE
11a

Stand with your feet hip-width apart.
Simultaneously push your hips back,
bend your knees slightly, and swing
your arms down to your sides. You'll
look like you're imitating the form of a
downhill skier. From there, forcefully
thrust your hips forward, straighten
your knees, and swing your arms
upward, so that you rise up on your
toes. Repeat the movement back and
forth quickly.

MAKE IT
HARDER
Jump off the floor
as you swing
upward.

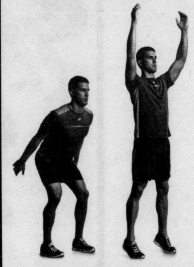

Plank to Rockback

EXERCISE
11b

Assume a pushup position, with your arms straight. Your body should form a straight line from your head to ankles. Without allowing your lower-back posture to change, bend your knees and push your hips backward. Then quickly "pull" yourself back to the starting position.

MAKE IT
HARDER

Instead of pulling yourself back to the starting position, pull yourself into the down position of a pushup. Then push into the rock-back position.

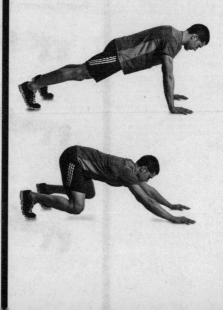

Plank Walkups

Start by getting into a pushup position, but bend your elbows and rest your weight on your forearms instead of your hands. Your body should form a straight line from your shoulders to your ankles. Now brace your core by contracting your abs as if you're about to be punched in the gut. Without allowing your body posture to change (don't let your hips sag!), place your right hand on the floor, then your left hand. Then push your body into the "up" position of a pushup. Now lower yourself back to your elbows into the plank position, by placing each elbow on the floor again. Repeat as many times as you can.

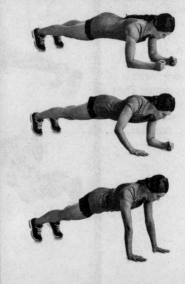

Skater Hops

EXERCISE

12 b

Stand on your right foot with your right knee slightly bent and your left foot slightly off the floor. Lower your body toward the floor, and then bound to your left by jumping off your right leg. Land on your left foot and bring your right foot behind your left as you reach toward the outside of your left foot with your right hand. Reverse the movement back toward the right, landing on your right foot.

Drop Squat

EXERCISE

13a

Stand with your feet together and toes forward. Jump your feet out to beyond shoulder-width as you push your hips back, bend your knees, and land in a squat position, your thighs nearly parallel to the floor. Immediately return to the starting position, jumping slightly and bringing your feet back together. Repeat.

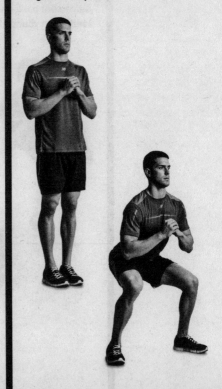

Triceps Pushup

EXERCISE
13b

MAKE IT
HARDER
Move your feet
farther back. You
could move them
just an inch or two,
or until your legs
are completely
straight (hardest).

Get down on all fours, with your hands
and knees on the floor. Now raise your
knees off the floor an inch or two. Bend
your elbows and lower your body until
your knees barely touch the floor. Push
back up and repeat. Keep your elbows
as close to your body as you can
throughout the movement.

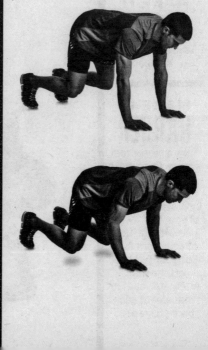

HOLD IT!
WORKOUTS

*You won't have to move a muscle in this
8-minute routine. Just maintain the
position and feel the fat burn away. Here's
how to do it: Simply hold the first exercise*

Prisoner Squat

EXERCISE
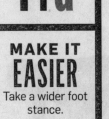

Place your fingers on the back of your
head, pull your elbows and shoulders
back, and stand with your feet
shoulder-width apart. Lower your body
as far as you can and hold that
position.

MAKE IT
EASIER

Take a wider foot
stance.

MAKE IT
HARDER

Take a closer foot
stance. Or to make
it even harder,
stagger your feet
by placing the toes
of your left foot in
line with the heel
of your right foot.
Lift your left heel
off the floor.
Alternate your foot
placement each
time you repeat.

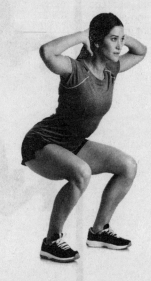

Bent-Knee Pushup Hold

EXERCISE

14b

Get down on all fours, with your hands and knees on the floor. Now raise your knees off the floor an inch or two and hold that position.

MAKE IT
HARDER

Raise one arm off the floor. (Alternate the arm each time you repeat.) You can also raise one leg off the floor, or raise your opposite leg and arm off the floor at the same time (hardest).

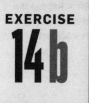

Single-Leg Squat

EXERCISE

15a

Stand on your left foot and hold your right foot off the floor. Push your hips back, bend your left knee, and lower your body as far as you comfortably can. Hold that position. Repeat the movement on your right leg. Try to lower a little farther each set.

Hip Hinge Plus Y

EXERCISE

15 b

Bend your knees slightly, push back your hips, and lower your torso while keeping your back straight. Now raise your arms at an angle in front of you until they're in line with your torso and form a Y position with your upper body. (The thumbside of your hands should be pointing toward the ceiling.) Hold that position.

Elevated Hip Extension

EXERCISE

16a

Lie on your back on the floor and place your heels on a bench or ottoman. Place your arms at an angle next your sides, palms down. Your legs should be completely straight. Now pull your toes toward your body, press your heels into the bench, and lift your hips off the floor until your body forms a straight line from shoulders to knees. Hold that position.

Side Plank

EXERCISE
16 b

Lie on your left side and prop your upper body up on your left forearm. Now brace your core, squeeze your glutes, and raise your hips until your body forms a straight line from shoulder to ankles. On your next set, switch sides.

MAKE IT
EASIER

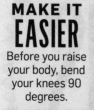

Before you raise your body, bend your knees 90 degrees.

MAKE IT
HARDER

Lift your top leg and hold it there.

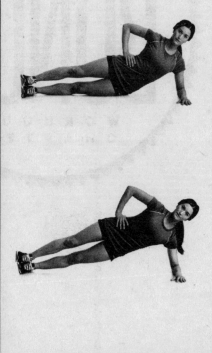

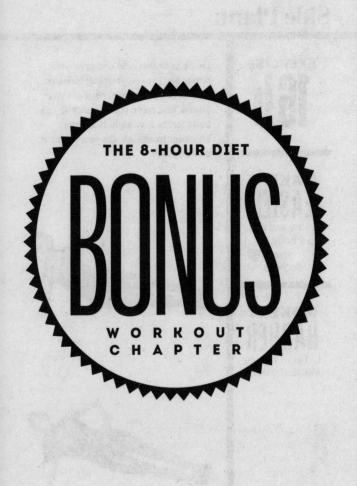

THE 8-HOUR DIET

BONUS

WORKOUT
CHAPTER

The 8-Minute Maximum Fitness Plan

Take your weight loss to a whole new level with these serious belly-blasting moves

Are you ready for the best workout of your life? This ultimate workout plan will tone your muscles and melt away fat faster than ever.

When you're on the 8-Hour Diet, you have a secret advantage over every other person you see pumping iron at the gym, stretching at the yoga studio, or sweating it out along the jogging trail. You're not working any harder than they are. But your body is building muscle and burning fat faster than theirs.

It's really kind of unfair.

But it's why you simply don't have to exercise as long or as vigorously as most folks do to get the physical benefits you're looking for. In just 8 minutes, you can set your body up for more lean, toned muscle and a greater all-day calorie burn. You just need the right workout. Fortunately, you've come to the right place.

8 Minutes to Lean

To get those muscle-building, fat-burning, 8-minute benefits, I turned to *Men's Health* fitness guru BJ Gaddour, a metabolic training expert and the man behind the bestselling fitness plan Speed Shred. He's doing more for people with eight DVDs than many in the fitness industry have done for them over the course of decades. BJ has an incredible physique, but he describes himself as a "former fatty"— and he has the photographic evidence to prove it. But what we didn't know until recently was that he only achieved part of his weight loss through devoted exercise. The rest: his own version of the 8-Hour Diet.

Just like Barack Obama, who experimented with fasting when he made his turn toward being a serious student at Columbia University, Gaddour assessed his life and wasn't happy with what he saw. And like Obama, Gaddour found he could dramatically improve his life by rethinking the way he ate. Fasting helped both of them turn it around—waistline, life goals, satisfaction, all of it.

Gaddour was first exposed to the idea of skipping meals at an early age by his father, Brahim Gaddour, who had emigrated to the United States from Tunisia as a young man. Gaddour the elder would fast in observance of the Muslim holy month of Ramadan. In addition to his religious goals, Brahim used his holy month as a weight-loss tool. But he didn't ever change his diet. He maintained that he simply couldn't eat as much in a single sitting during Ramadan because his stomach would shrink.

But it may have been because he exercised while fasting.

When Ramadan was scheduled during summer months, BJ watched in awe as his father challenged himself to work outdoors, to test himself in the sweltering heat. He found his father's sheer level of mental determination and dietary discipline awe inspiring. But he also noted how the physical element helped reinforce his father's observance of the fast.

It will vastly enrich yours, too.

Fasting and physical fitness began turning BJ Gaddour's life around at age 13, but he continued to struggle with weight gain into his adult years. When he finally committed to a pattern of eating for 8 hours a day and matching that with very targeted workout programs, he assumed the ultrafit form you see on him today—exhorting exercisers with his DVD series, or on his Web site StreamFIT.com. We're not saying you'll become a fitness guru yourself in just 8 minutes a day, but you can turbocharge your fat loss in that time—no time flat.

Gaddour has created an amazing 8-minute metabolic workout that you can do immediately upon waking, when you'd otherwise be eating breakfast. It will accelerate your fat-burning metabolism and provide the kind of focal point you need when Dunkin' Donuts beckons. Not only is this quick-hitter workout entirely equipment-free, you don't even have to join a gym. You can do all the moves at home, in a hotel room, in your office, indoors or outdoors, and they will burn 15 to 20 calories worth of body fat, or more, per minute. In your fasting state, you'll already be selectively burning body fat; this workout will torch even more. And on top of all that, it will target every muscle in your body to skyrocket your postworkout metabolism and keep your fat-and-calorie burn going.

This total body circuit can be as easy or as challenging as you want to make it—and you don't need to work hard to get remarkable results. Start with the simplest moves, and when they become familiar and easy, move to the more challenging variations Gaddour specifies. No matter what level you choose, you'll kick off an adrenaline release that will help chase stubborn fat from your belly, hips, and thighs. And in just 8 minutes you can deplete glycogen, the sugar stored in your skeletal muscles and liver, which forces your body to burn more fat for fuel at all other times, including rest periods and between workouts.

Ready to start? Set your watches: This will only take 0.133333 of an hour! (Did we mention it was 8 minutes long?)

The 8-Minute Workout at a Glance

★   Alternate between Workouts A, B, and C. So if you do A on Monday, try B on Wednesday and C on Friday or Saturday. Then back to A. You know the drill, right?

★   For the first 2 weeks, take a day of rest between workouts to recover. You'll quickly build up strength and endurance.

★   For weeks 3 and 4, perform a workout every day. Hey, it's only 8 minutes!

★   Start by performing each exercise within each circuit in the exact order listed for 30 seconds of work followed by 30 seconds of rest between exercises.

★   Each subsequent week, add 5 seconds of work and take away 5 seconds of rest until you end up converting this bodyweight circuit into a complex where you perform each move for 60 seconds with no rest between movements!

★   There is a built-in warm-up to each workout. The first move in each circuit mobilizes the often tight areas of the ankles, hips, and upper back.

EXERCISE	WORKOUT A	WORKOUT B	WORKOUT C
1	Spider Lunge/ Monkey Lunge Superset*	Predator Jack	Crab Walk
2	Ground-Zero Jump	Bear Crawl	Squat and Lunge Walk
3	Blast-Off Pushup	Kick-Through	Isometric Towel Row*
4	In and Out Squat	Power Step-Up/ Skater Jump Superset*	Low Box Runner/ Burpee Superset*
5-8	REPEAT EXERCISES 1–4		

*Switch moves at the halfway mark

Want to double or even triple the effectiveness of this workout?
★ For a 17-minute workout, employ a 1-minute rest and transition period after completing the 8-exercise circuit and do it once more.
★ For a 26-minute workout, employ a 1-minute rest and transition period after completing the 8-exercise circuit and do it two more times.

EXERCISE DESCRIPTIONS—AND BENEFITS!

Spider Lunge

WORKOUT

A

EXERCISE

1a

MAKE IT
EASIER

Perform slowly
and come onto
your back knee to
decrease loading
and instability
demands.

MAKE IT
HARDER

Increase the
speed of
movement.

WHY IT WORKS:

This is quite possibly one of the top moves
on the planet, especially for people who sit
at a desk all day. Its benefits include:

➤ Strengthening the shoulders.
➤ Stabilizing the spine.
➤ Mobilizing the hip flexors and groin.
➤ Teaching you how to move at the hips
and not the lumbar spine.

Advanced methods train fast-twitch fibers
and ballistic core stability.

HOW TO DO IT:

1 Assume a push-up position, loading
your palms with your hands directly
underneath your shoulders and
tightening your abs and glutes to form a
straight line from your head through
your heels. Now move your left foot so
you plant the heel just outside your left
hand without moving at your lower back.
2 Then explosively jump your hips up
and switch your legs midair so your right
foot lands just outside your right hand.
3 Keep switching back and forth and
repeat for time.

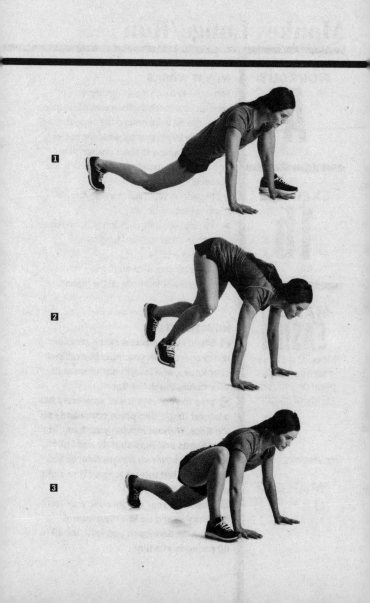

Monkey Lunge/Run

WORKOUT

A

EXERCISE

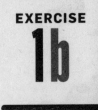

1b

MAKE IT
EASIER
Move at a slower, more controlled pace or with less range of motion.

WHY IT WORKS:

The monkey lunge is an amazing way to open up your inner thighs and hips. If you've ever suffered from groin pulls or tightness, then this move is exactly what the doctor ordered. Progress to the monkey run to skyrocket your metabolism and heart rate. Its benefits include:

➤ Mobilizing your hips in a side-to-side frontal plane of motion.

➤ Hitting your outer hip and glute muscles more than other forward lunging and crawling exercises.

➤ Smoking your shoulders more than probably any other move on the planet.

HOW TO DO IT:

1 Stand with your feet twice shoulder-width apart, push your hips back, bend your knees, and lower your torso until your hands touch the floor.

2 Step to your left, lower your body into a lateral lunge, and place both hands on the floor. Without moving your feet, lift your hands and hips slightly and shift your weight over your right foot, so you end up in a left lateral lunge. (Your right leg should straighten.)

3 Now shift your weight over your left foot, so you end up in a right lateral lunge. Alternate back and forth for 30 to 60 seconds at a time.

MAKE IT
HARDER

Turn it into a monkey shuffle run by simultaneously loading your hands, lifting your hips, and shuffling your feet side to side between right and left lunge positions.

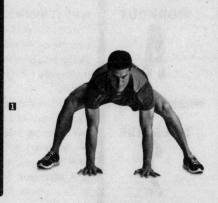

1

2

3

Ground-Zero Jump

WORKOUT

A

EXERCISE

2

MAKE IT
EASIER
Perform at a slower, more controlled speed.

MAKE IT
HARDER
Increase the speed of the movement and even go slightly airborne at the top.

WHY IT WORKS:

The ground-zero jump is basically an equipment-free version of a kettlebell skier swing and a lower-impact alternative to traditional jumping activities. Its benefits include:

➤ Working your whole body, especially your backside, and crushing calories like few moves can while sparing your joints.

➤ Targeting fast-twitch muscle fibers that have the biggest impact on your metabolism, athleticism, and heart rate.

➤ Strengthening your hips and core more than traditional cardio exercises such as running on the treadmill and plodding along on the elliptical.

HOW TO DO IT:

1 Stand with your feet hip-width apart with your toes pointing straight ahead and your knees "soft" and slightly flexed. This is the starting position. Now hinge back at your hips with a flat back and reach your arms back behind you like a downhill skier without squatting any farther.

2 Explosively push your hips forward to come to a full stand while swinging your arms. Increase the level of difficulty by rising up on your toes.

➤ Reverse the movement and repeat for 30 to 60 seconds at a time.

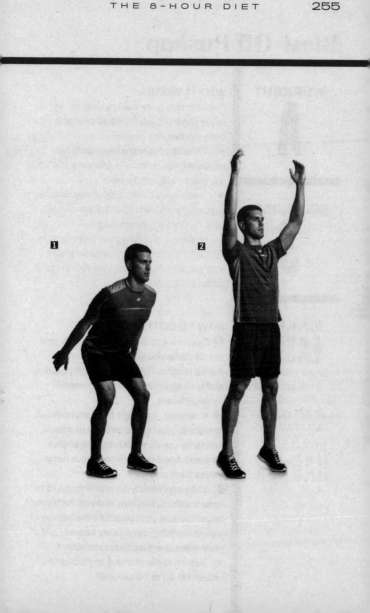

Blast-Off Pushup

WORKOUT

EXERCISE

3

MAKE IT EASIER

Don't lower into a full range of motion pushup or simply perform a pushup hold.

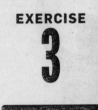

WHY IT WORKS:

This is probably the best pushup you've never done and will fry fat all over your body. Its benefits include:

➤ Working your entire lower body by mimicking the action of a sprinter's start or a lineman firing off the ball.

➤ Teaching you how to move at your hips explosively without moving at your lower back for unreal core stability.

➤ Pushing and pulling your upper body to sculpt a set of superhero shoulders from every angle while getting your heart rate through the roof!

HOW TO DO IT:

1 Assume a pushup position with your hands underneath your shoulders, palms loaded, tight abs and tight glutes, and a straight line from your head through heels.

2 Now push your hips back without moving at your lower back until your knees flex to about 90-degree angles and your head trails behind your hands. Pause for a count.

3 Then explosively extend through your knees, ankles, and hips and pull with your upper back as you lower into the bottom of a push-up with your elbows tucked tight at your sides to protect your shoulders.

➤ Return to the starting position and repeat for 30 to 60 seconds.

MAKE IT HARDER

Increase speed of movement or perform with your feet closer together, or even better, on one leg at a time.

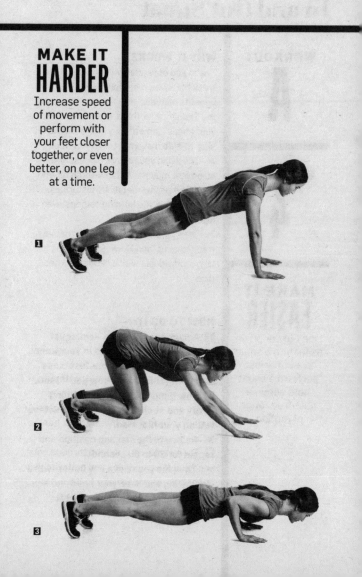

In and Out Squat

WORKOUT

EXERCISE

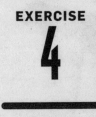

MAKE IT EASIER

Don't lower down as far into a squat or simply just perform a squat hold within a pain-free range of motion.

WHY IT WORKS:

The in and out squat will put you on the fast track to leaner, more toned legs. Its benefits include:

➤ Training your thigh muscles to stabilize your knees isometrically under a dynamic side-to-side movement with your feet.

➤ Involving your body's biggest and strongest muscles to blow-torch fat and cause a massive metabolic disturbance that will have you burning calories even after you stop doing it.

➤ Offering a lower-impact alternative to traditional up-and-down squat jumps for those individuals with a history of knee pain.

HOW TO DO IT:

1 Assume the athletic, semisquat position with triple bends in your knees, ankles, and hips with your feet close together. (This is also how you'll land.)

2 Now jump your feet out, landing softly and sticking it for a count, without letting your hips rise.

➤ Return to the starting position and repeat for 30 to 60 seconds.

➤ Imagine you're in a tiny house with a low ceiling and keep your head and hips down throughout the movement to protect your knees.

MAKE IT
HARDER
Increase speed of movement, perform the movement from a deeper squat position, or move in multiple directions.

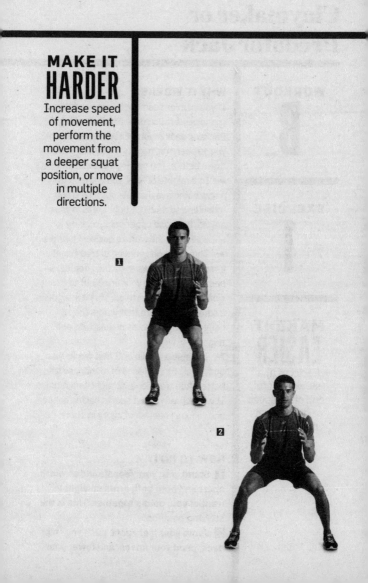

Claymaker or Predator Jack

WORKOUT B

EXERCISE 1

MAKE IT EASIER

Perform at a slower, more controlled speed or don't squat down as far.

WHY IT WORKS:

If you've ever seen the movie *Predator* or the celebration dance of Green Bay Packers' sack master Clay Matthews, then you've seen this mighty metabolic mobility move before. You can expect these benefits:

➤ In a minute or less, you'll fire up the nerve pathways that link your mind and muscles and mobilize tight areas in your ankles, hips, and upper back, making for quite possibly the world's quickest warm-up.

➤ This upgraded version of traditional jumping jacks is easier on the shoulders because you move your arms out to the sides instead of overhead, plus it integrates a squatting pattern that works the belly-busting muscles of your hips and thighs.

➤ It's also a cardio drill that works your body in all three planes of motion, so it's better than traditional straight-line running. It will actually boost sports performance and reduce your risk of injury in sport.

HOW TO DO IT:

1 Stand with your feet shoulder-width apart and hold both arms straight in front of you, palms together. This is the starting position.

2 Jump your feet apart, push your hips back, bend your knees, and lower your

MAKE IT
HARDER

Increase the speed of the movement or perform longer isometric holds at the bottom of the squat position.

body into a squat while pulling your arms apart and squeezing your shoulder blades together. (Your arms should be in line with or slightly behind your shoulders.)

3 Now shift your weight over your right leg and then your left leg before bringing it back to center and returning to the starting position.

➤ Repeat for 30 to 60 seconds, gradually increasing your speed and range of motion.

Bear Crawl

WORKOUT

B

EXERCISE

2

MAKE IT

EASIER

Perform slower and smaller crawling steps or simply hold the bear crawl position isometrically

WHY IT WORKS:

As they say, you must learn how to crawl before you can learn how to walk. And sometimes the best moves to burn fat are the ones we haven't done in a while (if ever), like crawling. Its benefits include:

➤ Being a foundational locomotion pattern that works your whole body with a specific emphasis on your shoulders and core.

➤ Building your quads much more than a regular straightlegged pushup position.

➤ Muscling up your upper body by moving on all fours instead of just your legs.

HOW TO DO IT:

1 Assume a bent-knee pushup position with your palms loaded with hands underneath your shoulders and your knees bent at 90-degree angles with your feet underneath your hips.

2 Now move your right hand and your left foot forward so that your opposite hand and foot are moving together in a contralateral pattern.

3 Switch sides and repeat for 30 to 60 seconds at a time.

MAKE IT
HARDER

Increase speed, distance traveled per step, or move backward or side-to-side. You can also perform bear crawls ipsilaterally with the same hand and foot moving together to increase the challenge.

1

2

3

Kick-Through

WORKOUT
B

EXERCISE
3

MAKE IT
EASIER

Move at a slower, more controlled pace, or sit on the outside of your hip as you move to each side.

WHY IT WORKS:

Many people consider the Turkish Get-Up, where you move from lying on your back to a full stand and back again, to be the ultimate total body exercise. That being said, it can be a tough and technical movement to perform, especially when in a state of fatigue. Enter my favorite metabolic version of a get-up called kick-through that will make you feel like you're literally break-dancing the fat off your belly. Its benefits include:

➤ Working single-arm shoulder strength and stability, much like a side plank.

➤ Teaching you how to move quickly and safely from a plank to bridge position and back.

➤ Hammering your hips, obliterating your obliques, and assaulting your abs in an almost criminal way.

HOW TO DO IT:

1 Assume a bent-knee push-up position with your palms loaded with hands underneath your shoulders and your knees bent at 90-degree angles with your feet underneath your hips.

2 Now kick your right leg underneath you as you roll onto your right hand to assume a one-arm, one-leg hip bridge position. Hold for a count.

MAKE IT
HARDER

Increase speed of motion or perform isometric holds in the one-arm, one-leg hip bridge position for 3 to 5 seconds at a time on each side. This move can also be performed forward to really increase the challenge.

➤ Reverse the movement, move to the other side, and repeat for 30 to 60 seconds at a time.

1

2

Power Step-Up

WORKOUT
B

EXERCISE
4a

MAKE IT
EASIER

Perform an eccentric step-up, taking 5 seconds to lower from the top to the bottom of the movement keep your knee and ankle aligned and your shin vertical.

WHY IT WORKS:

One of the best moves to build a better butt, boost metabolism, and ramp up fat loss is the power step-up. Not only is it a lower-impact version of lunge/split jumps that's easier on the knees, but it also trains both knee and hip extension, which is critical to proper running mechanics and overall athletic performance. Bottom line—the glute complex comprises the most metabolically active, calorie-burning tissue in your body. This means the more junk you've got in the trunk, the less fat you'll have everywhere else!

HOW TO DO IT:

1 Place your left foot onto a stable box/bench/step with your knee and ankle aligned, heel loaded and shin vertical.

2 Drive through your left heel and swing your arms overhead as you switch your legs midair, landing softly on the other side.

➤ Perform for 30 to 60 seconds at a time.

MAKE IT
HARDER
Increase the height of the box or step, increase the speed of movement or height of the jumps, or perform the jumps in a side-to-side fashion.

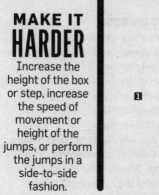

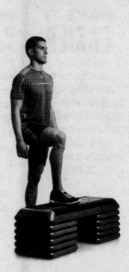

Skater Jump

WORKOUT

B

EXERCISE

4b

MAKE IT
EASIER
Perform at a slower, more controlled speed or place your back leg on the ground for extra support and stability when landing side to side.

WHY IT WORKS:

If you want to work your lungs and legs, then you simply cannot go wrong with the skater jump. Its benefits include:

➤ Heating up your hips and heart without as much stress on your knees as other forward-and-backward, up-and-down jumping drills create.

➤ Building wheels of steel by mimicking the movement of speed skaters on dry land.

➤ Training your hips in the often-neglected side-to-side frontal plane of motion to help reduce the risk of ACL tears when training or playing sports.

HOW TO DO IT:

1 Assume the athletic position with triple bends in your knees, ankles, and hips. (This is also how you'll land.) Push off your left leg and jump to the right leg, landing softly and sticking it for a count with your hips back and down.

2 Reverse the movement and repeat for 30 to 60 seconds, gradually increasing your speed and range of motion.

➤ Imagine you're in a tiny house with a low ceiling and keep your head and hips down throughout the movement to protect your knees.

MAKE IT
HARDER
Increase the speed of movement or the distance traveled or perform in multiple directions.

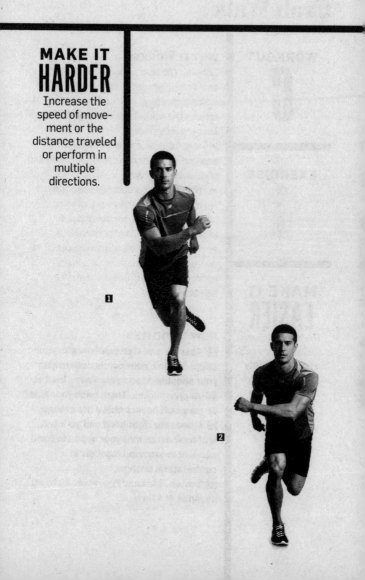

Crab Walk

WORKOUT

C

EXERCISE

1

MAKE IT
EASIER
Perform slower and smaller crab steps or simply hold the crab walk position isometrically.

WHY IT WORKS:

Consider the crab walk the opposite of the bear crawl. Where the bear crawl hits the entire frontside of your body, the crab walk attacks the whole back side of your body. Its benefits include:

➤ Mobilizing your hips and shoulders, especially important with all the typing and texting we do all day.

➤ Building your glutes and hamstrings, which are areas of the body that most people need to be more developed to improve both looks and performance.

➤ Targeting your triceps, which comprise two-thirds of the muscle mass in your upper arms, to amp up your arms in a serious way.

HOW TO DO IT:

1 Assume a seated position with your palms loaded, your hands underneath your shoulders, and your knees bent at 90-degree angles. Then, raise your hips so your butt hovers above the ground.

2 Move your right hand and your left foot forward so that your opposite hand and foot are moving together in a contralateral pattern.

3 Switch sides and repeat for 30 to 60 seconds at a time.

MAKE IT
HARDER

Increase speed of movement, distance traveled per step, or move backward or side-to-side. You can also perform crab walks from a high bridge position with a straight line from your head through hips.

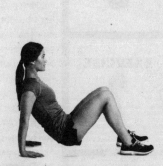

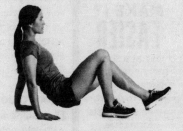

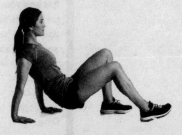

Squat-and-Lunge Walk

WORKOUT

C

EXERCISE

2

MAKE IT
EASIER

Move at a slower, more controlled pace or simply perform a staggered squat hold for a time.

WHY IT WORKS:

Most everyone knows that lunges and squats do both the legs and the body a great fitness service. However, integrating a walking pattern with both of these lower body builders is the quickest way to torch more calories and burn more fat. You can expect these benefits:

➤ The squat-and-lunge walk elevates your heart rate more than squats or lunges alone, resulting in more cardio conditioning and greater calorie burning.

➤ It hammers your quads but also teaches you how to shift your weight properly from hip to hip when in a staggered stance.

➤ The squat-and-lunge walk teaches you how to decelerate and absorb single-foot landings, which will boost running performance and reduce the risk of overtraining injuries like runner's knee.

HOW TO DO IT:

1 Assume a staggered squat position with your right leg forward with the heel flat and your left leg staggered behind on its toes so the toes are aligned with your right heel. Now push your hips back and down as far as you can while staying tall up top and stay there throughout the movement.

2 Walk forward, move to the other side and repeat for 30 to 60 seconds at a time.

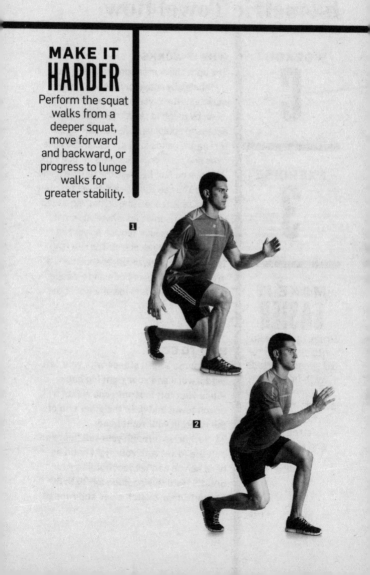

MAKE IT HARDER

Perform the squat walks from a deeper squat, move forward and backward, or progress to lunge walks for greater stability.

Isometric Towel Row

WORKOUT
C

EXERCISE
3

MAKE IT
EASIER

Break up the holds
into shorter 5 to
10 second periods
with brief 1 to
2 second rest
periods in between
to build up your
strength
and endurance
gradually.

WHY IT WORKS:

The upper back area comprises the most metabolically active, calorie-burning muscle tissue in your upper body. However, it can be tough to target this area without access to equipment like dumbbells and resistance bands for pulling exercises like rows and curls or pull-up bars for pull-ups. But have no fear because the terrible towel is here! You can use a beach towel to create manual resistance using something called overcoming isometrics where you create maximum muscular tension against an immovable force or object. The result? Improved posture, healthier shoulders, a more balanced upper body, and a V-taper that will turn heads in the office or at the beach.

HOW TO DO IT:

1 Assume a split stance with your left leg forward and your right leg back. Place your left foot onto one end of a beach towel and grab the other end of the towel in your right hand.

2 Now drive through your left heel and pull the towel with your right hand as hard as you can without holding your breath. Hold this position for 30 to 60 seconds, then switch sides and repeat.

MAKE IT
HARDER
Hold from a range
of motion that is
close to your rib-
cage and armpit
area to engage
your upper/
mid-back muscles
more fully.

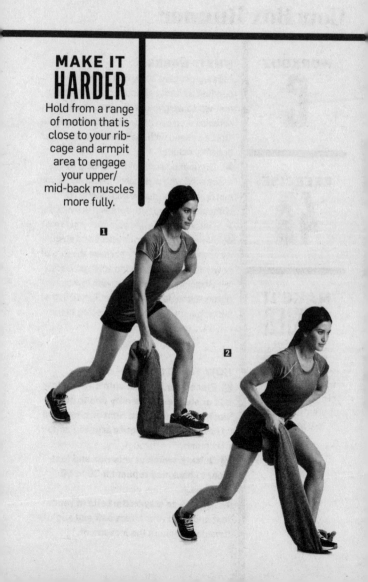

Low Box Runner

WORKOUT

C

EXERCISE

4a

MAKE IT
EASIER
Perform at a slower, more controlled tempo, focusing on nice, clean exchanges of your hands and feet.

WHY IT WORKS:

Although studies show that aerobic exercise just isn't that effective for producing real-world weight loss, the proper use of an aerobics step can be deadly to your body fat stores as seen with the low box runner. Its benefits include:

➤ Dissipating some of the landing forces associated with plyometric exercises so you can crank up the cardio and calorie burn without ending up with sore and achy joints.

➤ Getting you moving your feet and arms quickly to boost the bounciness and elasticity of your muscles and minimize the loss of power that comes with the aging process.

➤ Being great to combine with low box burpees (the next move in our Top 15 list) to add some total-body strengthening to the rapid fat-loss cardio chaos.

HOW TO DO IT:

1 Place your left foot onto a stable low box or step (even a sturdy phone book works here) with your right arm forward to resemble the opposite arm-leg action of running.

2 Quickly switch your hands and feet front to back and repeat for 30 to 60 seconds.

➤ Be sure to stay on the balls of your feet and keep your knees soft and slightly flexed throughout the movement.

MAKE IT
HARDER
Increase speed of movement, tap your feet for a couple counts before switching legs, or perform in multiple directions.

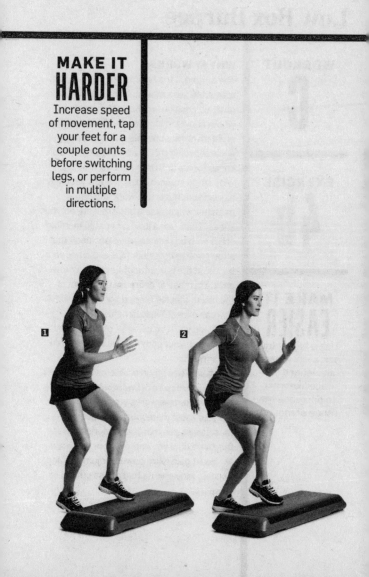

Low Box Burpee

WHY IT WORKS:

The burpee is the baddest exercise on the planet because moving from standing to a push-up position and back involves your whole body and blowtorches belly fat. The problem is, most people do it too quickly while rounding their backs and driving their knees forward. To remedy this, first use a wide sumo stance to better allow yourself to load your heels and work your glute muscles, which also takes pressure off your knees. Then, use a low box or step (aerobic steps with adjustable risers are ideal) that allows you to drop your hips and place your hands on the box without flexing your lower back. Increase or decrease the height of the box or step as needed and get to work! You can expect these benefits:

➤ Since you'll be using all of the biggest muscles in your body, the calorie burn will be fantastic.

➤ Usual knee strain problems are avoided by taking pressure off vulnerable hinges.

➤ This exercise works your glutes, which are your most metabolically active muscles, so you maximize calorie burn at the same time you improve your rear view.

➤ You'll gain extra power for jumping and twisting movements that are so critical to all sports.

MAKE IT
HARDER

Increase speed of movement, add a full push-up at the bottom of the movement, and/or add a jump onto the low box at the top of the move-ment. From there experiment with other variations.

HOW TO DO IT:

1 Assume a wide stance with your feet outside shoulder-width apart.

2 Keeping your back straight, load your heels and drop your hips until you can palm the box.

3 Then load your palms and jump your feet out into a push-up position, being sure to squeeze your glutes.

➤ Reverse the movement and repeat for 30 to 60 seconds.

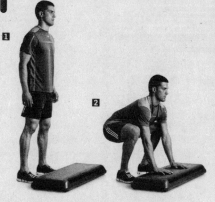

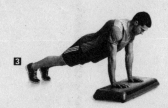

Index